Multiple Choice Questions in Gastroenterology

Other Examination Preparation Books Published by Petroc Press:

Black & Kelleher	*MCQs in Anaesthesiology*	1900603454
Chakravorty	*Visual Aids to the MRCP Examination*	0792388739
Edgell	*Preparing for MRCP Part II Cardiology*	0792388690
Green	*More MCQs for Finals*	079238928X
Green	*The MRCPsych Study Manual*	079238816X
Hogston	*MCQs for the MRCOG Part II*	0792388828
Kubba et al.	*MCQs for Memb. Faculty Family Planning Pt I*	1900603004
Levy & Riordan Eva	*MCQs in Optics and Refraction*	0792388356
Levy & Riordan Eva	*MCQs for the FRCOPHTH*	079238847X
Levy & Riordan Eva	*MCQs for the MRCOPHTH*	0792388488
Mokbel	*MCQs in Neurology*	0792388577
Mokbel	*MCQs in General Surgery*	1900603101
Mokbel	*MCQs in Applied Basic Sciences – 2nd edn*	0792388569
Mokbel	*Operative Techniques for the FRCS*	079238881X
Ross & Emmanuel	*MCQs in Medical Microbiology for MRCP*	0792388836
Ross & Emmanuel	*MCQs in Medical Microbiology and Infection*	0792388410
Ross & Emmanuel	*MCQs in Microbiology and Infection for FRCS*	1900603152
Rymer & Higham	*Preparing for the DRCOG*	0792388755
Sanderson *et al.*	*MCQs for the MRCP Part I*	0792388348
Sandler & Sandler	*MCQs in Cardiology for MRCP*	0792389999
Sandler & Sandler	*MCQs in Cardiology*	0792389387
Sandler & Sandler	*More MCQs in Cardiology for MRCP*	0792388402

Obtainable from all good booksellers or, in case of difficulty, from Plymbridge Distributors Limited, Plymbridge House, Estover Road, PLYMOUTH, Devon PL6 7PZ
Tel.   01752–202300
FAX   01752–202333

Multiple Choice Questions in Gastroenterology

Malcolm C. Bateson MD, FRCP, FRCP (Edinburgh)

Consultant and Specialist in Gastroenterology, General Hospital
Bishop Auckland

and

John G. Stephen MChir, FRCS

Consultant Surgeon, General Hospital
Bishop Auckland

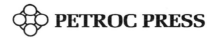 PETROC PRESS

Petroc Press, an imprint of Librapharm Limited

Distributors

Plymbridge Distributors Limited, Plymbridge House, Estover Road, Plymouth PL6 7PZ, UK

Published in the United Kingdom by Librapharm Limited, Gemini House, 162 Craven Road, Newbury, Berkshire RG14 5NR, UK

A catalogue record for this book is available from the British Library

ISBN 1 900603 40 3

Typeset by
Richard Powell Editorial and Production Services, Basingstoke, Hampshire
Printed and bound in the United Kingdom by
Hartnolls Limited, Bodmin, Cornwall

Contents

Introduction

These questions have been designed with various levels of difficulty so they should be suitable for clinical medical students, junior doctors, candidates for MRCP, and trainees in gastroenterology. Explanations of the answers are given.

Answers should only be indicated if candidates are completely or almost completely sure of the correct response.

Each correct answer scores 1 point but each wrong answer will lose marks, so it is best to leave blanks where there is serious uncertainty. Guessing can lose marks, and may lead to a low score even where many correct responses have been made in other questions.

This text should be an enjoyable self-teaching exercise. Do not be put off if you cannot answer all of the questions, since this is how learning occurs.

MCB

Bishop Auckland, 1996   JGS

1. Mouth, Pharynx and Oesophagus

Q1.1   Mouth ulcers are commoner in:

A. Diverticular disease
B. Coeliac disease
C. Solitary ulcer of rectum
D. Ulcerative colitis
E. Crohn's disease

Q1.2   Oral thrush is a frequent finding in:

A. Antibiotic therapy
B. Oral contraceptive use
C. Diabetes mellitus
D. HIV infection
E. Multiple sclerosis

Q1.3   Dental caries means increased likelihood of:

A. Gout
B. Subacute bacterial endocarditis
C. Alcoholism
D. Peptic ulcer
E. Dysphagia

Q1.4   An apparently enlarged tongue occurs in:

A. XIIth nerve palsy
B. Trisomy 21
C. Hypothyroidism
D. Duodenal ulcer
E. Coprolalia

Q1.5   A high arched palate is seen in:

A. Pseudoxanthoma elasticum
B. Wegener's granulomatosis
C. Cerebrotendinous xanthomatosis
D. Familial hypertriglyceridaemia
E. Marfan's syndrome

Q1.6   The presence of labial Herpes simplex means:

A. Very little
B. A recent cold
C. Shingles
D. Immune deficiency
E. Patient is on diclofenac

Q1.7   Crohn's disease affects the lips:

A. Rarely
B. Sometimes
C. Frequently
D. Never
E. Invariably

Q1.8   Presbyoesophagus:

A. Is a disease of young women
B. Is a normal variant of ageing
C. Causes oesophageal dilation with constriction rings
D. May be asymptomatic
E. Means the gullet is shorter

Q1.9   Parkinson's disease causes excess dribbling:

A. Because of increased salivation
B. Because of defective swallowing
C. Because patients are tremulous
D. Because of festination
E. Because of bradykinesia

Q1.10   In motor neurone disease:

A. True bulbar palsy is seen
B. Pseudobulbar palsy occurs
C. It is not possible to distinguish bulbar and pseudobulbar palsy
D. Swallowing can be normal
E. Sensory signs are uncommon

Q1.11 Post-cricoid carcinoma:

A. Always causes iron deficiency
B. Is not very common
C. May be missed by routine fibre-optic endoscopy
D. May be difficult to diagnose
E. Is managed by palliative intubation

Q1.12 Effective oesophageal stricture dilation may be achieved at endoscopy by:

A. Metoclopramide
B. Flexible bougies
C. Balloons
D. The endoscope itself
E. Retrograde cholangiography

Q1.13 Nicotinic acid deficiency causes:

A. Diarrhoea
B. Deafness
C. Dementia
D. Dermatitis
E. Dysmenorrhoea

Q1.14 Heartburn may be a symptom of:

A. Hiatus hernia
B. Gastro-oesophageal reflux
C. Peptic ulcer
D. Ischaemic heart disease
E. Rheumatic heart disease

Q1.15 A patient with no natural teeth or retained roots:

A. Never contracts sub-acute bacterial endocarditis
B. Needs less sedation for endoscopy
C. Is easier to endoscope
D. Will have a poor diet
E. Has reduced masticatory power

Q1.16 A 50-year-old man with new dyspepsia should:

A. Receive standard antacid therapy initially
B. Be investigated prior to any ulcer-healing therapy
C. Be referred to hospital
D. Be ignored because the condition is always self-limiting
E. Have an ECG

Q1.17 Gastro-oesophageal reflux can reliably be diagnosed by:

A. Symptoms
B. Biopsy histology of the gastro-oesophageal junction
C. Manometry
D. 24 hour pH monitoring
E. Bernstein test

Q1.18 Early gastric cancer is:

A. Rare outside Japan
B. Frequently cured
C. A precursor of advanced gastric cancer
D. Associated with drinking coffee
E. Associated with alcohol excess

Q1.19 A baby who becomes blue at feeding times may have as a reason:

A. Cyanotic heart disease
B. Exomphalos
C. Hiatus hernia
D. Tracheo-oesophageal fistula
E. Malrotation of the intestine

Q1.20 Drugs which have shown potential to improve mortality in gastrointestinal bleeding are:

A. Propranolol
B. Isosorbide dinitrate
C. Ranitidine
D. Somatostatin
E. Terlipressin

Q1.21 Measures to improve symptoms of oesophagitis include:

A. Sleeping propped up
B. Avoiding sport
C. Stopping smoking
D. Losing excess weight
E. Avoiding heavy meals

Q1.22 Oesophageal webs:

A. Should always be sought in iron deficiency anaemia
B. May be cured but not seen at endoscopy
C. Are best investigated by barium swallow
D. Are a pre-malignant condition
E. Are uncommon

Q1.23 Tracheo-oesophageal fistula is usually seen in:

A. Infants
B. Children
C. Young adults
D. Middle age
E. The elderly

Q1.24 An open safety pin in the oesophagus in an adult:

A. Should merely be observed
B. Needs immediate laparotomy
C. May be safely removed at endoscopy
D. Could perforate the aorta
E. Is radiolucent

Q1.25 Weight loss with oesophageal stricture:

A. Is eventually invariable
B. Means malignancy
C. Should be treated with home total parenteral nutrition
D. Should be more than 10 kg before therapy is required
E. Is often associated with regurgitation of food

Q1.26 Barrett's oesophagus is:

A. Absent squamous epithelium
B. Gastric metaplasia of the oesophagus
C. Intestinal metaplasia of the oesophagus
D. Pre-malignant
E. A variant of hiatus hernia

Q1.27 Sliding hiatus hernia is:

A. Very common
B. Sometimes fatal in adults
C. Usually asymptomatic
D. Difficult to diagnose with complete certainty
E. Associated with gastric carcinoma

Q1.28 The correct daily dose of cimetidine for healing reflux oesophagitis is:

A. 200 mg
B. 400 mg
C. 800 mg
D. 1600 mg
E. 3200 mg

Q1.29 Chest pain is likely to be oesophageal if:

A. It is external
B. It spreads to the arm
C. It causes dyspnoea
D. It is precipitated by food
E. It is relieved by antacid

Q1.30 Oesophageal cancer is especially common around:

A. American great lakes
B. Mediterranean
C. Caspian sea
D. Pacific coast of USA
E. Brighton marina

Q1.31 Oesophageal varices:

A. Are always present in cirrhosis
B. May be treated without laparotomy
C. Can be a cause of occult bleeding
D. May be effectively treated by injection
E. May lead to encephalopathy

Q1.32 With a Sengstaken tube:

A. The gastric balloon must be inflated before the oesophageal one
B. The oesophageal balloon must be inflated before the gastric one
C. Both balloons should be inflated together
D. The oesophageal balloon should not be inflated for more than 24 hours
E. Blood should be aspirated from the oesophageal balloon

Q1.33 The following are proven to be useful in prolonging life in oesophageal varices:

A. Portacaval anastomosis
B. Propranolol
C. Nitrate therapy
D. Ranitidine
E. Prednisolone

Q1.34 Chagas' disease is caused by:

A. Viruses
B. Bacteria
C. Chlamydia
D. Fungi
E. Protozoa

Q1.35 An isotope swallow test can prove the presence of:

A. Gastro-oesophageal reflux
B. Dysmotility
C. Presbyoesophagus
D. Oesophagitis
E. Achalasia

Q1.36 VII nerve palsy occurs in:

A. Mumps
B. Parotid calculi
C. Carcinoma of the parotid
D. Sialectasis
E. Amyotrophic lateral sclerosis

Q1.37 The following are important in the management of perforated oesophagus:

A. Surgery
B. Nasogastric suction
C. IV ranitidine
D. Antibiotics
E. Autopsy

Q1.38 Biopsy histology in oesophagitis shows:

A. Hyperkeratosis
B. Plentiful mitoses
C. Thickening of the surface epithelium
D. Deepening of the rete pegs
E. Superficial ulceration

Q1.39 Reflux oesophagitis is often associated with:

A. Obesity
B. Cigarette smoking
C. Hiatus hernia
D. Atropinic drugs
E. Manual work

Q1.40 Dysphagia may be caused by:

A. Cerebrovascular disease
B. Alcohol excess
C. Peptic stricture
D. Stomach cancer
E. Pharyngeal pouch

Q1.41 The commonest site for cancer in men world-wide is:

A. Lung
B. Liver
C. Stomach
D. Large bowel
E. Pancreas

Q1.42 Professional singers and actors are especially prone to:

A. Glossitis
B. Cheilitis
C. Angular stomatitis
D. Aphthous ulceration
E. Vocal nodules

Q1.43 Parotitis is seen in:

A. Viral infections
B. Vegetarians
C. Vestibular neuronitis
D. Alcoholism
E. Clostridium infections

Q1.44 Fat digestion commences with enzymes produced in:

A. The cheeks
B. The pharynx
C. The stomach
D. The small intestine
E. The pancreas

Q1.45 Peppermint is especially useful treatment for:

A. Flatus
B. Constipation
C. Functional bowel disease
D. Dyspepsia
E. Diarrhoea

Q1.46 Pigmentation of the lips or buccal mucosa can be seen in:

A. Cushing's syndrome
B. Addison's disease
C. Vogt-Koyanagi syndrome
D. Peutz-Jegher syndrome
E. Marfan's syndrome

Q1.47 Tylosis is hyperkeratosis of the palms and soles. It may be:

A. Familial
B. Innocent
C. Linked with oesophageal carcinoma
D. Linked with tuberculosis
E. Cured by phototherapy

Q1.48 Disease of the oesophagus is seen in:

A. Scleroderma
B. Polymyalgia rheumatica
C. Polyarteritis nodosa
D. Self poisoning
E. Hiccups

Q1.49 Achalasia causes abnormalities detected by:

A. Barium swallow
B. Chest radiography
C. Isotope swallow
D. Endoscopy
E. Manometry

Q1.50 The best test of the presence of oesophagitis is:

A. Biopsy at the gastro-oesophageal junction
B. Endoscopy
C. Manometry
D. Barium swallow
E. Glycerine trinitrate

Q1.51 Oesophageal spasm responds to:

A. Glycerine trinitrate
B. Nifedipine
C. Hydralazine
D. Captopril
E. Minoxidil

Q1.52 Peptic oesophagitis is seen mainly in the following part:

A. Distal
B. Middle
C. Proximal
D. All of the above
E. None of the above

Q1.53 The following are helpful in diagnosis of rupture of the oesophagus:

A. Chest X-ray
B. Iodine contrast swallow
C. Rigid oesophagoscopy
D. ECG
E. Nasogastric intubation

Q1.54 Oesophageal carcinoma can be effectively treated by:

A. Conventional external radiotherapy
B. Chemotherapy
C. Open surgery
D. Palliative intubation
E. NdYAG laser therapy

Answers to Section 1

Q1.1
A. False
B. True
C. False
D. True
E. True
There may be an immune mechanism for these associations.

Q1.2
A. True
B. False
C. True
D. True
E. False
Antibiotic therapy will permit fungal overgrowth by suppressing competition. Diabetes and AIDS suppress immunity.

Q1.3
A. False
B. True
C. True
D. False
E. True
The mechanisms are different. Caries will be a focus of streptococci in SBE and will make mastication difficult. Alcoholics tend to neglect themselves.

Q1.4
A. False
B. True
C. True
D. False
E. False
The tongue will atrophy in XII nerve palsy and is unaffected in duodenal ulcer and coprolalia.

Q1.5
A. **False**
B. **False**
C. **False**
D. **False**
E. **True**

The high arched palate is actually part of the diagnostic definition of Marfan's syndrome.

Q1.6
A. **True**
B. **False**
C. **False**
D. **False**
E. **False**

Most of us will get cold sores from time to time.

Q1.7
A. **True**
B. **False**
C. **False**
D. **False**
E. **False**

Oral Crohn's disease probably affects 1% or less of patients.

Q1.8
A. **False**
B. **True**
C. **True**
D. **True**
E. **False**

This is a not uncommon finding in older patients.

Q1.9
A. **False**
B. **True**
C. **False**
D. **False**
E. **False**

Parkinsonian patients do not produce excess saliva but are unable to swallow it.

Q1.10
A. True
B. True
C. True
D. True
E. True

Q1.11
A. False
B. True
C. True
D. True
E. False

Post-cricoid carcinoma is uncommon and may present with iron deficiency, but not always. It occurs in a region that is very difficult to visualise with the gastroscope, and the area is not really suitable for palliative intubation.

Q1.12
A. False
B. True
C. True
D. True
E. False

Passage of any instrument through an oesophageal stricture tends to improve swallowing. Though wider dilation achieves better results the risks are higher.

Q1.13
A. True
B. False
C. True
D. True
E. False

Diarrhoea, altered mental state and a photosensitive skin rash are a classic presentation of severe nicotinic acid deficiency.

Q1.14
A. False
B. True
C. True
D. True
E. False

Though hiatus hernia may be associated with gastro-oesophageal reflux, it is the presence of the latter which causes the heartburn.

Q1.15
A. False
B. False
C. True
D. False
E. True
Gastroscopy is certainly easier in the absence of natural teeth.

Q1.16
A. True
B. True
C. True
D. False
E. False
Over the age of 40–45 the presence of organic disease including carcinoma of the oesophagus and stomach is greater. It is safest to gastroscope these patients before any therapy which might interfere with results.

Q1.17
A. False
B. False
C. False
D. True
E. False
Though tedious to perform, 24 hour pH monitoring is the best test for gastro-oesophageal reflux symptoms. The Bernstein acid perfusion tests are unreliable, manometry is difficult to standardise and interpret, and biopsy at the gastro-oesophageal junction usually shows some changes which must be regarded as normal.

Q1.18
A. False
B. True
C. True
D. False
E. True
Though the Japanese have the biggest experience of early gastric carcinoma because of high prevalence, the same disease occurs else-where. It is well worthwhile treating aggressively because it can be cured, unlike advanced gastric cancer. Cigarette smoking and alcohol excess are both associated.

Q1.19
A. False
B. False
C. False
D. True
E. False

This is the classic presentation of tracheo-oesophageal fistula. A baby with cyanotic heart disease will be blue all the time.

Q1.20
A. True
B. True
C. True
D. True
E. True

Propranolol, nitrates, somatostatin and terlipressin have all been shown to be useful in oesophageal varices. Intravenous ranitidine is useful in prevention of bleeding from stress ulcers in seriously ill patients.

Q1.21
A. True
B. False
C. True
D. True
E. True

These are all measures which should avoid gastro-oesophageal reflux.

Q1.22
A. False
B. True
C. True
D. True
E. False

Barium contrast is the best way of demonstrating oesophageal web, but it is not completely reliable, and they can be missed. Some resistance to gastroscopy is often explained by the presence of an oesophageal web.

Q1.23
A. True
B. False
C. False
D. False
E. False

Congenital tracheo-oesophageal fistulas are usually diagnosed in infancy. Secondary fistulas may occur later in life.

Q1.24
A. **False**
B. **False**
C. **True**
D. **True**
E. **False**
Endoscopic removal is often the safest plan.

Q1.25
A. **True**
B. **False**
C. **False**
D. **False**
E. **True**
Oesophageal strictures should respond to dilatation therapy and are usually benign. Those strictures which are malignant can be managed by dilatation, laser therapy, palliative intubation, external beam and intra-cavity radiation, and surgery.

Q1.26
A. **False**
B. **True**
C. **False**
D. **True**
E. **False**
Gastric metaplasia of the oesophagus is a response to reflux disease and is sometimes pre-malignant.

Q1.27
A. **True**
B. **False**
C. **True**
D. **True**
E. **False**
There is no absolutely unequivocal way of diagnosing hiatus hernia, which is often asymptomatic anyway.

Q1.28
A. False
B. False
C. False
D. True
E. False

Oesophagitis is less amenable to treatment than peptic ulcers and really vigorous acid suppression is required.

Q1.29
A. False
B. False
C. False
D. True
E. True

The other characteristics are those of angina.

Q1.30
A. False
B. False
C. True
D. False
E. False

This interesting observation is definite but not explained.

Q1.31
A. False
B. True
C. True
D. True
E. False

Standard treatment of oesophageal varices includes Sengstaken tube, injection sclerotherapy, banding, terlipressin and propranolol. Bleeding leads to high protein content of the gut which precipitates encephalopathy.

Q1.32
A. True
B. False
C. False
D. True
E. False

The gastric balloon is the anchor which avoids displacement, which may be dangerous. Prolonged inflation of the oesophageal balloon can cause local ulceration in the oesophagus.

Q1.33
A. **False**
B. **False**
C. **False**
D. **False**
E. **False**
Though treatments A to C are effective they do not definitely prolong life.

Q1.34
A. **False**
B. **False**
C. **False**
D. **False**
E. **True**
This is South American trypanosomiasis.

Q1.35
A. **True**
B. **True**
C. **False**
D. **False**
E. **True**
In reflux disease contrast returns from the stomach to the oesophagus either spontaneously or on provocation. In dysmotility oesophageal clearing is delayed and in achalasia there is complete stasis of contrast in the oesophagus.

Q1.36
A. **False**
B. **False**
C. **True**
D. **False**
E. **False**
Local pressure or invasion are probably the crucial mechanisms.

Q1.37
A. True
B. True
C. True
D. True
E. False

Most cases of iatrogenic oesophageal perforation are best managed without surgery.

Q1.38
A. False
B. False
C. True
D. True
E. True

These comprise the histological definition of oesophagitis.

Q1.39
A. True
B. True
C. True
D. True
E. False

Occupation is not known to be important.

Q1.40
A. True
B. False
C. True
D. True
E. True

Q1.41
A. False
B. True
C. False
D. False
E. False

Hepatitis B related primary liver cancer is currently commonest, though smoking related cancers are on the increase in the developing world.

Q1.42
A. False
B. False
C. False
D. False
E. True

Over-use of the voice causes nodules on the vocal cords which may require removal.

Q1.43
A. True
B. False
C. False
D. True
E. False

Mumps and alcohol abuse are common causes of parotitis.

Q1.44
A. False
B. True
C. False
D. False
E. False

Lipase is quite widely produced though the pancreas is the most prolific source.

Q1.45
A. False
B. False
C. True
D. True
E. False

Peppermint oil capsules are effective in irritable bowel syndrome and are much more concentrated than the mints that people suck for in-digestion.

Q1.46
A. False
B. True
C. False
D. True
E. False

In Addison's disease pigmentation may also occur in scars and in Peutz-Jegher's syndrome it is seen around the fingers.

Q1.47
A. True
B. True
C. True
D. False
E. False

In some cases tylosis is linked with oesophageal carcinoma, but often it is not.

Q1.48
A. True
B. False
C. False
D. True
E. False

Scleroderma causes local fibrotic infiltration of the oesophagus and reflux disease. Self-poisoning (classically with bleach) causes strictures.

Q1.49
A. True
B. True
C. True
D. True
E. True

All tests tend to be abnormal in true achalasia.

Q1.50
A. False
B. True
C. False
D. False
E. False

Oesophagitis is a superficial problem best identified under direct vision. Any biopsies should be at least 2 cm proximal to the gastro-oesophageal junction.

Q1.51
A. True
B. True

C. **True**
D. **False**
E. **False**

Q1.52
A. **True**
B. **False**
C. **False**
D. **False**
E. **False**
Gastro-oesophageal reflux will affect the distal oesophagus first.

Q1.53
A. **True**
B. **True**
C. **False**
D. **False**
E. **False**
Oesophageal perforation will lead to pleural effusion and air in the mediastinum, pleural cavity and sub-cutaneously. Water soluble contrast radiology will identify the size and position of the perforation.

Q1.54
A. **True**
B. **False**
C. **True**
D. **True**
E. **True**
Chemotherapy has not been shown to be useful overall.

2. Stomach and Duodenum

Q2.1 The best duration of treatment to ensure 90% duodenal ulcer healing with H2 receptor antagonist is:

A. 1 week
B. 2 weeks
C. 4 weeks
D. 8 weeks
E. 1 year

Q2.2 Effective ulcer treatment which works without any action on gastric acid secretion is:

A. Lactulose
B. Aluminium hydroxide
C. Sucralfate
D. Lactitol
E. Magnesium trisilicate

Q2.3 Antacid therapy relieves symptoms:

A. Rapidly
B. By complete neutralisation of gastric acid
C. By eradicating *Helicobacter pylori*
D. Indefinitely
E. By protecting the mucosa from acid

Q2.4 The best management for a 10-year-old with prolonged abdominal pain is:

A. Immediate endoscopy
B. Referral to a paediatric gastroenterologist
C. Cimetidine 400 mg
D. General Practitioner care
E. Lithium

Q2.5 The best management for a 70-year-old with haematemesis is:

A. Hospital admission
B. Ferrous sulphate
C. Ranitidine 300 mg at night
D. Observation at home
E. Sengstaken tube

Q2.6   What are the most suitable antacids to achieve relief of symptoms without side-effects:

A. Baking soda
B. Calcium carbonate
C. Hydrotalcite
D. Magnesium and aluminium hydroxides
E. Milk

Q2.7   Pernicious anaemia is associated with:

A. Auto-immune gastritis
B. Dyspepsia
C. Thyroid disease
D. Liver disease
E. Neuropathy

Q2.8   Important causes of gastritis are:

A. Eating curries
B. Smoking cigarettes
C. Drinking excess alcohol
D. Chewing gum
E. Drinking "cola"

Q2.9   Basal and peak acid output are most important in the diagnosis of:

A. Duodenal ulcer
B. Gastrinoma
C. Gastric ulcer
D. Gastric carcinoma
E. Rickets

Q2.10 Gastric atony can occur in:

A. Motor neurone disease
B. Marfan's syndrome
C. Friedreich's ataxia
D. Diabetes insipidus
E. Diabetes mellitus

Q2.11 Gastroenteritis is normally best treated by:

A. Hydration alone
B. Anti-emetics
C. Anti-diarrhoeals
D. Antibiotics
E. Lactulose

Q2.12 Hunger pains are:

A. Normal
B. More frequent in peptic ulcer
C. Sometimes seen in carcinoma
D. Rapidly relieved by food
E. Always pathological

Q2.13 Gastric surgery may be followed by:

A. Osteomalacia
B. Weight loss
C. Pulmonary tuberculosis
D. Gallstones
E. Gastric cancer

Q2.14 Gastric cancer is becoming:

A. Very common
B. A bit more common
C. No commoner and no rarer
D. Less common
E. Very rare

Q2.15 Gastric carcinoma is especially common in:

A. Mexico city
B. Qatar
C. Barnsley
D. Tokyo
E. Zurich

Q2.16 The success of peptic ulcer surgery can be judged by:

A. Insulin test meal
B. Sham feeding
C. Pre- and post-operative pentagastrin test meals
D. Symptoms
E. Gastric pH monitoring

Q2.17 Gastrinoma:

A. Often lies in the pancreas
B. Can be treated by ranitidine 300 mg at night
C. Causes diarrhoea
D. May become malignant
E. Is rare

Q2.18 *Helicobacter pylori* bacteria:

A. Live in gastric acid
B. Adhere to the gastric mucosa in an alkaline layer
C. Are never seen in healthy people
D. Can be simply identified in the endoscopy room by their urease activity
E. Are associated with peptic ulcer relapse

Q2.19 The stomach is sometimes involved in:

A. Coeliac disease
B. Lymphoma
C. Crohn's disease
D. Alactasia
E. Barrett's oesophagus

Q2.20 Satisfactory management for metastatic gastric carcinoma may include:

A. Vagotomy
B. Gastric radiotherapy
C. 5-fluorouracil
D. Cyclosporin A
E. Prednisolone

Q2.21 Taste is governed by:

A. I cranial nerve
B. III cranial nerve
C. VII cranial nerve
D. IX cranial nerve
E. XI cranial nerve

Q2.22 Atropinic treatment for peptic disease is limited by:

A. High prevalence of side-effects in effective doses
B. Expense
C. Problem of induction of gastro-oesophageal reflux
D. Adverse effects in complete heartblock
E. Low efficacy

Q2.23 Prostaglandin analogues heal peptic ulcers but:

A. Are slow to take effect
B. Have some action on gastric acid
C. Have an unusually high relapse rate
D. Cause diarrhoea
E. Are unlikely to be drugs of first choice

Q2.24 After peptic ulcers have healed with anti-acid therapy they recur:

A. Never
B. Sometimes
C. Usually
D. Almost always in the first year
E. Inevitably

Q2.25 Duodenal ulcer is commoner in:

A. Women
B. Social classes I and II
C. Asian British
D. Doctors
E. None of the above

Q2.26 Duodenal ulcer can cause:

A. Haemorrhage
B. Constipation
C. Perforation
D. Gastric outflow obstruction
E. Blackouts

Q2.27 Chagas' disease may be suspected if a patient has:

A. Constipation
B. Dysphagia
C. Heart failure
D. Jaundice
E. Reflux oesophagitis

Q2.28 Refractory dyspepsia may respond to:

A. Ursodeoxycholic acid
B. Lithocholic acid
C. Metoclopramide
D. Haloperidol
E. Prednisolone

Q2.29 Active peptic ulcers contra-indicate treatment with:

A. Aspirin
B. Steroids
C. Oral contraceptives
D. Warfarin
E. Paracetamol

Q2.30 A patient with a third episode of gastrointestinal haemorrhage from an unknown site should be offered first:

A. Early endoscopy
B. Barium radiology
C. Laparotomy
D. Intravenous acid-suppressing therapy
E. A Sengstaken tube

Q2.31 Results of medical therapy have made elective surgery for peptic ulcer:

A. Obsolete
B. Less common
C. More common
D. Inevitable
E. None of the above

Q2.32 The hospital mortality from bleeding peptic ulcer is:

A. 1%
B. 3%
C. 5%
D. 10%
E. 20%

Q2.33 Non-steroidal anti-inflammatory drugs are:

A. The best treatment in osteo-arthritis
B. Responsible for an increasing death rate from peptic ulcer haemorrhage in the elderly
C. Useful treatment for soft tissue injuries and acute gout
D. Safer than aspirin
E. About equivalent with each other in effect

Q2.34 Signs suggestive of malignancy in a gastric ulcer are:

A. Small size
B. Rolled edges
C. Refractoriness to healing therapy
D. Occurrence on the proximal greater curve
E. Young age of patient

Q2.35 Weight loss and amenorrhoea are seen in:

A. Thyrotoxicosis
B. Anorexia nervosa
C. Ovarian carcinoma
D. Fibroids
E. Stein–Leventhal syndrome

Q2.36 Menetrier's disease:

A. Affects the small bowel
B. Causes protein loss
C. May be associated with achlorhydria
D. Responds well to H_2 receptor antagonist therapy
E. Is frequently refractory to therapy

Q2.37 Modern treatments of gastric ulcer include:

A. Antacids
B. Carbenoxolone
C. Deglycyrrhizinised liquorice
D. Propantheline
E. Milk diet

Q2.38 Vomiting in the elderly is best treated with:

A. Prochloperazine
B. Chlorpromazine
C. Diazepam
D. Metoclopramide
E. Doperidone

Q2.39 Body mass index is measured by:

A. Weight $\div$ height
B. Weight^2 $\div$ height
C. Weight $\div$ height^2
D. Weight^2 $\div$ height^2
E. Weight^3 $\div$ height

Q2.40 The causes of dyspepsia include:

A. Irritable bowel syndrome
B. Peptic ulcer
C. Gallstones
D. Diverticular disease
E. Carcinoma

Q2.41 Reliable symptoms of duodenal ulcer are:

A. Fat intolerance
B. Radiation of pain to back
C. Night waking
D. Precipitation by alcohol
E. Early morning retching

Q2.42 Tests which are useful in diagnosing pernicious anaemia include:

A. 2-part Schilling test
B. Barium meal
C. Endoscopy
D. Gastric biopsy
E. Tissue antibody screen

Q2.43 A Bezoar is:

A. A polyp in the stomach
B. A congenital abnormality
C. A fibre ball
D. A variety of peptic ulcer
E. A type of gastrectomy

Q2.44 The standard operation for a benign gastric ulcer is:

A. Proximal gastric vagotomy
B. Selective vagotomy and pyloroplasty
C. Truncal vagotomy and antrectomy
D. Partial gastrectomy and gastro-duodenostomy
E. Partial gastrectomy and gastroenterostomy

Q2.45 Medical therapy for benign gastric ulcer:

A. Always works
B. Usually works
C. Sometimes works
D. Often fails
E. Always fails

Q2.46 Peak acid output is

A. The highest pH level in 24 hours
B. The amount of acid produced after a meal
C. The maximum response to pentagastrin stimulation
D. Is always abnormal in peptic ulcer
E. Reduced after vagotomy

Q2.47 True pyloric stenosis:

A. Causes vomiting in infancy
B. Results from duodenal ulceration in adults
C. Requires ultrasonograpy for diagnosis
D. Follows gastric annular carcinoma
E. Is usually treated by vagotomy and pyloroplasty

Q2.48 Hiatus hernia:

A. Invariably causes symptoms
B. Requires surgery more frequently in children than adults
C. Is usually only important when oesophageal reflux occurs
D. Is recognisable at endoscopy by a 'B' ring in the stomach at the level of the diaphragm
E. Is generally present in patients with heartburn

Q2.49 A stomach involved in linitis plastica:

A. May look normal at endoscopy
B. May look normal on barium meal
C. Carries a very poor prognosis
D. May yield normal histology on forceps biopsy
E. Requires emergency total gastrectomy

Q2.50 *Helicobacter pylori* infections are detected by:

A. Gastric pH monitoring
B. Gastric biopsy and microscopy
C. Gastric biopsy and culture
D. Gastric biopsy and urease activity
E. Serology

Q2.51 Ulcer-healing drugs which work by blocking the action of histamine on the stomach include:

A. Omeprazole
B. Terfenadine
C. Famotidine
D. Azatadine
E. Nizatidine

Q2.52 Fibre-optic upper digestive endoscopy:

A. Is less accurate than video endoscopy
B. Is superior to barium meal examination
C. Replaces the need for small bowel biopsy capsules in coeliac disease
D. Has no mortality
E. Usually requires IV sedation which may be reversed with flumazenil

Q2.53 Iron deficiency anaemia in rheumatoid arthritis:

A. Often responds to iron therapy
B. Often responds to ulcer healing drugs
C. May reflect the effect of NSAID therapy
D. May be refractory to all treatment
E. Is rare

Q2.54 Mortality in patients with gastrointestinal haemorrhage:

A. Is low under 65 years
B. Is definitely reduced by vigorous antacid therapy
C. Relates mainly to associated diseases
D. Is higher in oesophageal variceal bleeding
E. Is higher in Mallory–Weiss tears

Q2.55 Useful actions of lansoprazole include:

A. Rapid healing of peptic ulcers
B. Suppression of *H. pylori*
C. Control of symptoms of gastrinoma
D. Inhibition of gastric histamine receptors
E. Reduction of gastro-oesophageal reflux

Answers to Section 2

Q2.1
A. False
B. False
C. False
D. True
E. False
Though shorter treatment periods are frequently used, only 6 to 8 weeks therapy will reliably heal 90% or more of duodenal ulcers.

Q2.2
A. False
B. False
C. True
D. False
E. False
Sucralfate functions as a mucosal protective.

Q2.3
A. True
B. False
C. False
D. False
E. False
If antacid therapy works, it works quickly but needs to be given by repeated doses.

Q2.4
A. False
B. True
C. False
D. True
E. False
Children need careful evaluation, but invasive investigation and blind treatment are not usually appropriate.

Q2.5
A. True
B. False
C. False
D. False
E. False

Significant gastrointestinal bleeding may require transfusion and certainly will need investigation.

Q2.6
A. False
B. False
C. True
D. True
E. False

Sodium bicarbonate is a rapidly effective antacid but can cause vomiting and hypokalaemia. The high calcium load in calcium antacids and milk may have adverse effects.

Q2.7
A. True
B. True
C. True
D. False
E. True

There is no strong link between pernicious anaemia and even autoimmune liver disease.

Q2.8
A. False
B. True
C. True
D. False
E. False

Tobacco and alcohol excess are linked with gastritis. Curry, chewing gum and "cola" are the habitual diet of many normals.

Q2.9
A. False
B. True
C. False
D. False
E. False

Classically basal and peak acid output after pentagastrin stimulation are the same in gastrinoma. These tests do not contribute to the diagnosis of the other conditions.

Q2.10
A. **False**
B. **False**
C. **False**
D. **False**
E. **True**

Motility disorders in diabetes mellitus are common and often difficult to treat.

Q2.11
A. **True**
B. **False**
C. **False**
D. **False**
E. **False**

Overall best results are obtained by allowing the disease to run its course while maintaining hydration. However, specific antibiotic treatment may be helpful in salmonella, campylobacter or amoebic infections.

Q2.12
A. **True**
B. **True**
C. **True**
D. **True**
E. **False**

Symptoms are not a reliable indicator of diagnosis.

Q2.13
A. **True**
B. **True**
C. **True**
D. **True**
E. **True**

Partial gastrectomy is associated with many health problems in its own right.

Q2.14
A. **False**
B. **False**

C. False
D. True
E. False
The prevalence of gastric cancer has been falling for many years.

Q2.15
A. False
B. False
C. False
D. True
E. False
Japan has the highest prevalence of gastric carcinoma in the world, probably from a combination of genetic and geographical reasons.

Q2.16
A. True
B. True
C. True
D. True
E. True
All of these techniques have been used in assessment of peptic ulcer surgery, but are very little required now.

Q2.17
A. True
B. False
C. True
D. True
E. True
Though famous gastrinoma is very uncommon indeed. Some patients can be managed by proton pump inhibitor therapy.

Q2.18
A. False
B. True
C. False
D. True
E. True
50% of the world's population carry *Helicobacter pylori*, which lives closely applied to the gastric epithelium under the mucus layer. It is a combination of gastric acid and *Helicobacter pylori* together with other factors which is responsible for peptic ulcer disease. Urease test may be rapidly positive but requires review the following morning.

Q2.19
A. **False**
B. **True**
C. **True**
D. **False**
E. **False**
Gastric lymphoma (MALToma) is a discrete problem strongly linked with
H. pylori infection.

Q2.20
A. **False**
B. **False**
C. **True**
D. **False**
E. **False**
Chemotherapy is disappointing, but is worth considering especially in
younger patients.

Q2.21
A. **True**
B. **False**
C. **True**
D. **True**
E. **False**
The taste buds are supplied by the VIIth and IXth cranial nerves. but much of
the sensation of taste is actually smell mediated through the olfactory nerve.

Q2.22
A. **True**
B. **False**
C. **True**
D. **False**
E. **False**
Though atropinics have an effect on gastric secretion, this is not really
useful in practical therapy.

Q2.23
A. **False**
B. **True**
C. **False**
D. **True**
E. **True**

Prostaglandin analogues probably work mainly via their weak gastric acid suppression activity, but diarrhoea is a major limitation to effective treatment.

Q2.24
A. False
B. False
C. True
D. False
E. False

Peptic ulcers must be regarded as a chronic relapsing condition unless *H. pylori* is eradicated.

Q2.25
A. False
B. False
C. False
D. False
E. True

Q2.26
A. True
B. False
C. True
D. True
E. False

These are the classic complications of duodenal ulcer disease.

Q2.27
A. True
B. True
C. True
D. False
E. False

This interesting condition is only a problem in Latin America.

Q2.28
A. True
B. False
C. True
D. False
E. False

Pro-kinetic therapy may be useful especially in reflux symptoms. The mechanism of improvement after bile acid therapy is not clear and this is an expensive option.

Q2.29
A. True
B. True
C. False
D. True
E. False

It should now be possible to eradicate peptic ulcer disease, so these therapies can then safely be given.

Q2.30
A. True
B. False
C. False
D. False
E. False

Early diagnosis is the only effective way to plan management.

Q2.31
A. False
B. True
C. False
D. False
E. False

Occasional patients still need elective surgery.

Q2.32
A. False
B. False
C. False
D. True
E. False

Though a wide range of figures is sometimes quoted, 10% is the closest approximation to overall experience.

Q2.33
A. False
B. True
C. True

D. **False**
E. **True**

These drugs and aspirin require cautious use to protect the GI tract.

Q2.34
A. **False**
B. **True**
C. **True**
D. **True**
E. **False**

Fortunately most gastric ulcers are benign, but histology and surveillance to prove healing are both important to avoid missing cancers.

Q2.35
A. **True**
B. **True**
C. **False**
D. **False**
E. **False**

These are classic presentations.

Q2.36
A. **False**
B. **True**
C. **True**
D. **False**
E. **True**

If patients are positive for *Helicobacter pylori* specific eradication therapy has been proposed.

Q2.37
A. **True**
B. **False**
C. **False**
D. **False**
E. **False**

Antacids will give symptomatic relief. The other drugs and the milk diet are obsolete.

Q2.38
A. **False**
B. **False**
C. **False**

D. True
E. True
It is best to use specific anti-emetic therapy to avoid sedation and Parkinsonian effects.

Q2.39
A. False
B. False
C. True
D. False
E. False
Body mass index (BMI or Quelet's Index) is calculated from weight in kilograms divided by the square of the height in metres. The ideal is 20–25. Over 30 is obese and over 40 is morbidly obese.

Q2.40
A. True
B. True
C. False
D. False
E. True
Gallstones should not be blamed for simple dyspepsia.

Q2.41
A. False
B. True
C. True
D. False
E. False
Radiation to the back and night waking are the only symptoms in this grouping specifically linked to duodenal ulcer.

Q2.42
A. True
B. False
C. False
D. True
E. True
If an anaemic patient with a low B12 carries intrinsic factor antibody the diagnosis is pernicious anaemia. If not, a Schilling test is needed to prove the diagnosis. Gastric biopsy will provide some support.

Q2.43
A. False
B. False
C. True
D. False
E. False
These are commonly formed by hair or vegetable fibres.

Q2.44
A. False
B. False
C. False
D. True
E. False
If surgery is required then partial gastrectomy, excising the ulcer, and a gastro-duodenostomy give best results.

Q2.45
A. False
B. True
C. False
D. False
E. False
Therapy may need to be prolonged.

Q2.46
A. False
B. False
C. True
D. False
E. True

Q2.47
A. True
B. False
C. False
D. True
E. False
Duodenal ulcer may cause gastric outflow obstruction but this is a post-pyloric problem.

Q2.48

A. **False**
B. **True**
C. **True**
D. **True**
E. **False**

The important question in hiatus hernia is whether gastro-oesophageal reflux occurs and is causing significant problems.

Q2.49

A. **True**
B. **False**
C. **True**
D. **True**
E. **False**

This sub-mucosal tumour may be missed at gastroscopy, but barium meal appearances are very characteristic.

Q2.50

A. **False**
B. **True**
C. **True**
D. **True**
E. **True**

Direct urease testing is the first line procedure where endoscopy is being performed anyway. Serology yields equivalent results and is useful in epidemiology. Urea breath tests are also helpful and are mainly used to demonstrate eradication after therapy.

Q2.51

A. **False**
B. **False**
C. **True**
D. **False**
E. **True**

Omeprazole is a proton pump inhibitor, and terfenadine and azatidine are H1 receptor antagonists.

Q2.52

A. **False**
B. **True**
C. **True**

D. False
E. False
Video and fibre-optic gastroscopy yields equivalent results and are more reliable than barium meal examination overall. Procedures may be conducted without sedation and this is often safer. Complications and deaths often relate to cardio-respiratory problems in the elderly.

Q2.53
A. True
B. True
C. True
D. True
E. False
Though normochromic normocytic anaemias refractory to iron are characteristic of rheumatoid arthritis, GI blood loss related to drug therapy is a common problem also.

Q2.54
A. True
B. False
C. True
D. True
E. False
Mallory–Weiss tears are usually self-limiting. No anti-acid therapy has been proved to be effective in in-patients.

Q2.55
A. True
B. True
C. True
D. False
E. True
Proton pump inhibitors are now first line treatment for peptic disease and may conveniently be combined with antibiotics in anti-*Helicobacter* regimens.

3. Nutrition, Absorption and the Intestine

Q3.1 **Retching without vomiting before breakfast may indicate:**

A. Gallstones
B. Pancreatitis
C. Alcoholism
D. Anorexia nervosa
E. Pregnancy

Q3.2 **Bottled mineral water is healthier than British tap water because:**

A. It often has bubbles
B. It has a greater mineral content
C. It contains trace elements absent from normal diets
D. There are no germs in it
E. It comes from spas

Q3.3 **Fat intolerance is an important symptom in patients with:**

A. Gallstones
B. Cirrhosis
C. Colon cancer
D. Hypertriglyceridaemia
E. Coeliac disease

Q3.4 **Appetite is governed by:**

A. A sense of smell
B. Centres in the thalamus
C. Emotional well-being
D. Social class
E. Physical exercise

Q3.5 **The following are common causes of food poisoning:**

A. *Staphylococcus epidermidis*
B. *Salmonella* species
C. *Serratia marescens*
D. *Clostridium perfringens*
E. *Bacillus cereus*

Q3.6   The following are causes of dysentery:

A. *Shigella* species
B. *Campylobacter* species
C. *Entamoeba histolytica*
D. Pathogenic escherichia
E. *Diphyllobothrium latum*

Q3.7   Giardiasis is:

A. Only seen in children
B. Associated with IgA deficiency
C. More frequent in travellers to Russia
D. Usually cured by metronidazole
E. A worm infestation

Q3.8   Failure to culture pathogens in acute diarrhoeal illness:

A. Is rare
B. Means the illness is not infective
C. Could indicate rotavirus infection in children
D. Requires combined broad-spectrum anti-microbial therapy
E. Is common

Q3.9   Modern therapy for worm infestation:

A. Is less toxic than previous treatment
B. Has a very satisfactory success rate
C. Avoids the need for purgation
D. Often requires only a single dose
E. Is metronidazole

Q3.10 In food allergy the following types of food are especially suspect:

A. Cheese
B. Rice
C. Eggs
D. Lamb
E. Chocolate

Q3.11 Vegans are:

A. People who do not eat meat
B. People who do not eat animal products at all
C. Protected from cancer of the pancreas
D. At risk for vitamin B_{12} deficiency
E. Sometimes Rastafarians

Q3.12 Anaemia with a low corpuscular haemoglobin and small cells may be seen in:

A. The post-gastrectomy state
B. Pernicious anaemia
C. Thalassaemia
D. Alcoholism
E. Occult bleeding

Q3.13 Serum B12 levels are:

A. Low in malabsorption
B. High in liver disease
C. High after hydroxocobalamin therapy
D. Normal in dementia
E. Usually abnormal in coeliac disease

Q3.14 Of all the patients seen in gastroenterology clinics with abdominal pain how many are not found on investigation to have an organic disease:

A. 2%
B. 10%
C. 25%
D. 50%
E. 75%

Q3.15 Typhoid:

A. Is caused by salmonella
B. Is effectively treated with chloramphenicol
C. May be recognised early by the profuse watery diarrhoea
D. Does not cause raised temperature
E. Needs admission to an intensive therapy unit

Q3.16 Foods to avoid in coeliac disease are:

A. Wheat
B. Oats
C. Maize
D. Rye
E. Barley

Q3.17 Dermatitis herpetiformis is sometimes:

A. Linked with coeliac disease
B. Gluten-sensitive
C. Diagnosed by skin immunohistochemistry
D. Present without a blistering rash
E. Familial

Q3.18 To diagnose Crohn's disease properly patients must have:

A. Pain
B. Diarrhoea
C. Perineal sepsis
D. A small bowel enema
E. A family history

Q3.19 A body mass index of 29:

A. Is normal
B. Is plump
C. Will shorten life
D. Is common
E. Is desirable

Q3.20 Bulimia is a condition where:

A. Starvation and vomiting alternate
B. Weight gain is usual
C. An organic cause is present
D. Psychiatric help is indicated
E. Hair loss is invariable

Q3.21 Intravenous feeding is:

A. Better than enteral feeding
B. Must be given before all major surgery
C. Has no serious complications
D. Expensive
E. Should be considered in anorexia nervosa

Q3.22 Human life can be sustained by water alone for:

A. 3 days
B. 7 days
C. 10 days
D. 6 weeks
E. 12 weeks

Q3.23 Food intolerance is:

A. Always allergic
B. Often associated with atopy
C. Uncommon in Caucasians
D. Best determined by exclusion diets
E. Associated with schizophrenia

Q3.24 Measurement of the following in breath is clinically relevant:

A. Nitrogen
B. Methane
C. Carbon dioxide
D. Hydrogen
E. Hydrogen sulphide

Q3.25 Black stools can be caused by:

A. Iron therapy
B. Guinness
C. Bismuth
D. Liquorice
E. Altered blood

Q3.26 A child with coeliac disease who ceases to thrive:

A. Is probably not keeping to the diet
B. Could have a lymphoma
C. Is likely to have primary biliary cirrhosis
D. Is intolerant of rice
E. May grow up short

Q3.27 Crohn's disease:

A. Frequently affects the terminal ileum
B. May be multicentre
C. May only affect the colon
D. Is rapidly fatal
E. Affects 1% of the population

Q3.28 A patient with acute right lower quadrant abdominal pain could have:

A. Acute appendicitis
B. Crohn's disease
C. No definable illness
D. Diverticular disease
E. Caecal carcinoma

Q3.29 Tests for alactasia include:

A. Lactose tolerance test
B. Galactose tolerance test
C. Glucose tolerance test
D. Breath hydrogen
E. Drinking milk

Q3.30 Small bowel bacterial overgrowth:

A. Can be determined by $[^{14}C]$-glycocholate breath test
B. Should respond to antibiotic therapy
C. Can be associated with diverticulosis
D. Causes increased breath hydrogen
E. May cause constipation

Q3.31 Fat malabsorption

A. Always causes diarrhoea
B. Is never seen in obesity
C. Is easily diagnosed without stool collection
D. Is mild in pancreatic insufficiency
E. Is seen after Polya gastrectomy

Q3.32 Major causes of steatorrhoea are:

A. Oesophageal stricture
B. Gastric surgery
C. Coeliac disease
D. Pancreatic insufficiency
E. Caecal carcinoma

Q3.33 First-line management for symptomatic small bowel Crohn's disease includes:

A. Prednisolone
B. Azathioprine
C. Levamisole
D. Sulphapyridine
E. Surgery

Q3.34 After resection of segments of Crohn's disease the annual relapse rate is approximately:

A. 1%
B. 3%
C. 5%
D. 10%
E. 25%

Q3.35 In India small bowel granulomatous disease is likely to be:

A. Leprosy
B. Sarcoidosis
C. Crohn's disease
D. Tuberculosis
E. Silicosis

Q3.36 In a child or young adult obscure intestinal bleeding is likely to be from:

A. Angiodysplasia of colon
B. Idiopathic thrombocytopenia
C. Meckel's diverticulum
D. Christmas disease
E. Polycythaemia

Q3.37 Obscure intestinal bleeding is sometimes a feature of:

A. Pseudoxanthoma elasticum
B. Osler–Weber–Rendu syndrome
C. Warfarin treatment
D. Paracetamol treatment
E. Familial combined hyperlipidaemia

Q3.38 Pertechnetate isotope scanning will localise:

A. Gastrinoma
B. Gastric heterotopia
C. Duodenal ulcers
D. Vipoma
E. Somatostatinoma

Q3.39 In a combined 2-part Schilling test malabsorption usually shows:

A. Normal excretion of both isotopes
B. High excretion of one isotope
C. High excretion of both isotopes
D. Low excretion of one isotope
E. Low excretion of both isotopes

Q3.40 Intestinal gas is largely:

A. Swallowed air
B. Excreted CO_2
C. Bacterial methane
D. Hydrogen
E. Hydrogen sulphide

Q3.41 Multiple fluid levels in the small intestine suggest:

A. Water intoxication
B. Crohn's disease
C. Intestinal obstruction
D. Gastric hypersecretion
E. Pyloric stenosis

Q3.42 Disease of the small intestine can cause diarrhoea because of:

A. Fat malabsorption
B. Bile acid malabsorption
C. Altered motility
D. Bacterial overgrowth
E. Villous atrophy

Q3.43 Essential components of a healthy human diet include:

A. Minerals
B. Vitamins
C. Protein
D. Fat
E. Meat

Q3.44 Abnormality of triolein breath test indicates steatorrhoea and is indicated by:

A. Breath hydrogen greater than 20 ppm
B. Breath $^{14}CO_2$ less than 0.4% mmol CO_2/kg
C. Breath methane greater than 1%
D. Dyspnoea
E. None of the above

Q3.45 Pneumatosis coli:

A. Is large bowel gas gangrene
B. Is invariably fatal
C. Responds to rectal nitrogen therapy
D. Responds to inhaled oxygen
E. Is uncommon

Q3.46 Constipation could be:

A. The result of a faulty diet
B. Associated with steatorrhoea
C. Caused by African trypanosomiasis
D. Hirschsprung's disease
E. Cured by magnesium hydroxide

Q3.47 Alternating diarrhoea and constipation suggest:

A. Pyloric stenosis
B. Psychotic illness
C. Irritable bowel syndrome
D. Adrenal insufficiency
E. Coeliac disease

Q3.48 Painless diarrhoea and weight loss may be a feature of:

A. Crohn's disease
B. Ulcerative colitis
C. Thyrotoxicosis
D. Primary biliary cirrhosis
E. Infective hepatitis type A

Q3.49 Obscure frank rectal bleeding is seen in:

A. Angiokeratoma corporis diffusum
B. Angiodysplasia
C. Allergy to food
D. α-1-antitrypsin deficiency
E. Lymphangiectasia

Q3.50 A young woman with eosinophilic gastroenteritis:

A. Will always have definite trigger foods
B. Should be investigated by small bowel biopsy
C. May require steroid therapy if illness does not settle
D. Could benefit from an exclusion diet
E. May respond to oral sodium cromoglycate

Q3.51 Purgative abuse:

A. Causes hypokalaemia
B. Causes hypocalcaemia
C. Leads to constipation
D. Sometimes shows as pigmentation in the colon
E. Always responds to medical advice to desist

Q3.52 The commonest age for presentation of ulcerative colitis is:

A. 10–20 years
B. 20–40 years
C. 40–60 years
D. 60–80 years
E. Over 80 years

Q3.53 Non-specific ulcerative jejunoileitis:

A. Is often severe coeliac disease
B. Does not always respond to gluten exclusion
C. Is harmless
D. May require steroid therapy
E. May cause perforation

Q3.54 Absorption of nitrogen from the intestine is most efficient in the form of:

A. Amino acids
B. Dipeptides
C. Polypeptides
D. Protein
E. Creatinine phosphokinase

Q3.55 Carbohydrate is absorbed as:

A. Monosaccharide
B. Disaccharide
C. Glycans
D. Cellulose
E. Porphyrins

Q3.56 Fats are absorbed in the form of:

A. Fatty acids
B. Monoglycerides
C. Diglycerides
D. Triglycerides
E. Prostaglandins

Q3.57 Intestinal water absorption is enhanced by:

A. Sugar
B. High roughage diet
C. Diuretic therapy
D. Starch
E. Carbonated beverages

Q3.58 Irritable bowel syndrome is most commonly seen in:

A. Young men
B. Young women
C. Middle-aged men
D. Middle-aged women
E. Elderly women

Q3.59 High fibre diet in irritable bowel syndrome:

A. Improves pain
B. Improves diarrhoea
C. Improves constipation
D. Is quite ineffective
E. Is harmless

Q3.60 Mental testing in usually abnormal in irritable bowel syndrome and the useful drugs for prolonged therapy are:

A. Diazepam
B. Propranolol
C. Chlorpropamide
D. Mianserin
E. Lithium

Q3.61 Coeliac disease carries a high prevalence of:

A. HLA - B_5
B. HLA - B_8
C. HLA - B_{27}
D. HLA - B_{35}
E. HLA - B_{52}

Q3.62 The cause of coeliac disease was found in:

A. 1914
B. 1936
C. 1944
D. 1963
E. 1979

Q3.63 In simple coeliac disease the immune globulin IgA is:

A. High or normal
B. Normal
C. Low or normal
D. Absent
E. Macroaggregated

Q3.64 Vomiting can cause:

A. Alkalosis
B. Acidosis
C. Pneumonitis
D. Haemorrhage
E. Surgical emphysema

Q3.65 The following dietary fats are protective to health:

A. Saturated
B. Monounsaturated
C. Polyunsaturated
D. Marine omega triglycerides
E. Palm oil

Q3.66 A history in gastrointestinal assessment should include:

A. Allergy questioning
B. Alcohol consumption
C. Tobacco usage
D. Drug therapy in past
E. Weight change

Answers to Section 3

Q3.1
A. False
B. False
C. True
D. False
E. True

Alcoholism characteristically causes "dry heaves" and morning nausea and sickness are often seen in pregnancy.

Q3.2
A. False
B. False
C. False
D. False
E. False

There is no overall advantage in mineral water.

Q3.3
A. False
B. False
C. False
D. False
E. False

Fat intolerance is not a very helpful clue as to the cause of symptoms.

Q3.4
A. True
B. True
C. True
D. False
E. True

Q3.5
A. False
B. True
C. False

D. True
E. True
The other organisms are not enteric pathogens.

Q3.6
A. True
B. True
C. True
D. True
E. False
Diphyllobothrium is the fish tapeworm.

Q3.7
A. False
B. True
C. True
D. True
E. False
Giardia is a protozoan and can affect adults. There are endemic areas and immune deficiency predisposes to infection. Metronidazole is the best treatment.

Q3.8
A. False
B. True
C. True
D. False
E. False
It is often difficult to pinpoint the cause of infective diarrhoeas.

Q3.9
A. True
B. True
C. True
D. True
E. False
Mebendazole and niclosamide are useful.

Q3.10
A. True
B. False
C. True

D. False
E. True
To test for food allergy patients are often started on a diet of lamb, rice and pears as these are hypo-allergenic foods, and then gradually suspect foods may be introduced.

Q3.11
A. False
B. True
C. False
D. True
E. True
Vegans do not eat meat or dairy products and consequently are at risk from B_{12} deficiency.

Q3.12
A. True
B. True
C. True
D. False
E. True
All of these conditions may be associated with iron deficiency anaemia. Alcoholics may be anaemic but characteristically have macrocytosis.

Q3.13
A. True
B. True
C. True
D. True
E. False
Displacement of liver stores may elevate serum B_{12} levels in liver disease, and hydroxycobalamin injections will also give high levels. Malabsorption may cause low levels, but coeliac disease is characterised by anaemias of iron and folate deficiency.

Q3.14
A. False
B. False
C. False
D. True
E. False

Many of the symptoms investigated cannot be shown to have a physical cause, though this doesn't necessarily make patients easier to look after.

Q3.15
A. True
B. True
C. False
D. False
E. False

Typhoid is enteric fever. It responds to a variety of antibiotics including ciprofloxacin, amoxycillin and chloramphenicol.

Q3.16
A. True
B. True
C. False
D. True
E. True

Maize is known to be harmless in coeliac disease and this is important as it is the cereal present in cornflakes. There is still a question mark over the safety of oats.

Q3.17
A. True
B. True
C. True
D. True
E. True

Q3.18
A. False
B. False
C. False
D. True
E. False

Small bowel radiology is important because this part of the intestine is preferentially affected in Crohn's disease. All the other features, though they may be present, are inconstant.

Q3.19
A. False
B. True

C. False
D. True
E. False

It is only over a body mass indexes of 40 that life expectancy is shortened markedly, though lesser degrees of obesity may affect physical health.

Q3.20
A. True
B. False
C. False
D. True
E. False

This condition can be very difficult to diagnose because the self-induced cause of symptoms is often concealed.

Q3.21
A. False
B. False
C. False
D. True
E. False

Though intravenous feeding is often necessary, alternatives should always be considered first. It may actually re-enforce problems in anorexia nervosa.

Q3.22
A. False
B. False
C. False
D. True
E. False

After 6 weeks irreversible break-down of essential body proteins begins.

Q3.23
A. False
B. True
C. True
D. True
E. False

Food intolerance is often difficult to pinpoint convincingly. It rarely seems to occur in those patients who consider they have it.

Q3.24

A. **False**
B. **False**
C. **True**
D. **True**
E. **False**

A variety of breath tests are available using labelled carbon dioxide, e.g. the triolein breath test. Breath hydrogen can be used in tests of absorption and dysmotility.

Q3.25

A. **True**
B. **True**
C. **True**
D. **True**
E. **True**

There are many dietary causes of black stool and testing for occult blood can be useful in evaluating them.

Q3.26

A. **True**
B. **True**
C. **False**
D. **False**
E. **True**

Failure to adhere to the diet is the most likely problem.

Q3.27

A. **True**
B. **True**
C. **True**
D. **False**
E. **False**

Crohn's disease may affect various parts of the GI tract and occurs in 1:1000 or less of the population.

Q3.28

A. **True**
B. **True**
C. **True**
D. **False**
E. **True**

Diverticular disease would normally present with left-sided abdominal pain.

Q3.29
A. True
B. False
C. False
D. True
E. True

Precipitation of symptoms by drinking a litre of milk is a simple screening test.

Q3.30
A. True
B. True
C. True
D. True
E. False

This condition is usually found in investigation of diarrhoea and malabsorption.

Q3.31
A. False
B. False
C. True
D. False
E. True

The triolein breath test is a convenient means of assessment of steatorrhoea. Fat malabsorption is usually marked or severe in significant pancreatic insufficiency.

Q3.32
A. False
B. True
C. True
D. True
E. False

Q3.33
A. True
B. True
C. False
D. False
E. True

The immuno-stimulant levamisole has adverse effects which limit its use. Sulphapyridine is merely an old-fashioned sulphonamide.

Q3.34

A. **False**
B. **False**
C. **False**
D. **True**
E. **False**

An average period free of relapse of 7 years is a realistic expectation.

Q3.35

A. **False**
B. **False**
C. **False**
D. **True**
E. **False**

Tuberculosis is common and Crohn's disease is rare in India.

Q3.36

A. **False**
B. **False**
C. **True**
D. **False**
E. **False**

This can be demonstrated by pertechnetate scanning which will document the ectopic gastric mucosa.

Q3.37

A. **True**
B. **True**
C. **True**
D. **False**
E. **False**

Q3.38

A. **False**
B. **True**
C. **False**
D. **False**
E. **False**

Q3.39

A. **False**
B. **False**

C. False
D. False
E. True
In pernicious anaemia isotope bound to intrinsic factor should be absorbed and excreted normally.

Q3.40
A. True
B. False
C. False
D. False
E. False

Q3.41
A. False
B. False
C. True
D. False
E. False
The presence of a few fluid levels may be normal.

Q3.42
A. True
B. True
C. True
D. True
E. True
All of these causes need to be considered in a diagnostic work-up.

Q3.43
A. True
B. True
C. True
D. True
E. False
Vegetarians are perfectly healthy.

Q3.44
A. False
B. True
C. False

D. False
E. False
This test depends on radio-labelling of the carbon in oleic acid which is excreted in breath.

Q3.45
A. False
B. False
C. False
D. True
E. True
This unusual condition is associated with lung emphysema and causes multiple gas bubbles in the wall of the large bowel.

Q3.46
A. True
B. True
C. False
D. True
E. True
Most constipation is caused by a low roughage diet. It may occur in fat malabsorption. Hirschsprung's disease is caused by lack of the myenteric nerve plexus and magnesium hydroxide is a purgative.

Q3.47
A. False
B. False
C. True
D. False
E. False
This is one of the major characteristics of irritable bowel syndrome.

Q3.48
A. True
B. True
C. True
D. True
E. True
Many other conditions may present in this way too.

Q3.49
A. False
B. True

C. **False**
D. **False**
E. **False**
Angiodysplasia frequently is found in the right colon by colonoscopy.

Q3.50
A. **False**
B. **True**
C. **True**
D. **True**
E. **True**
This condition is difficult to diagnose accurately and treatment is unsatisfactory. Peripheral blood eosinophilia is an important clue.

Q3.51
A. **True**
B. **False**
C. **True**
D. **True**
E. **False**
Serious purgative abuse is often concealed.

Q3.52
A. **False**
B. **True**
C. **False**
D. **False**
E. **False**
Inflammatory bowel disease may present at any age but the third and fourth decades of life are the most likely.

Q3.53
A. **True**
B. **True**
C. **False**
D. **True**
E. **True**
This condition may make patients very ill indeed.

Q3.54
A. **False**
B. **True**
C. **False**

D. False
E. False
The theoretical advantage of dipeptides has not really justified their routine inclusion in artificial feeds, which commonly contain polypeptides and whole protein.

Q3.55
A. True
B. False
C. False
D. False
E. False
Apart from simple sugars, carbohydrates require digestion before absorption.

Q3.56
A. True
B. True
C. False
D. False
E. False
Immediately after absorption fats are re-synthesised into triglycerides.

Q3.57
A. True
B. False
C. False
D. True
E. False
These are components of rehydration mixtures for diarrhoeal illness.

Q3.58
A. False
B. True
C. False
D. True
E. False
Despite the heavy female preponderance, men are certainly not immune from this condition.

Q3.59
A. False
B. False

C. **True**
D. **False**
E. **True**
Results of high roughage treatment in all irritable bowel cases has been disappointing, and it should be reserved for those with predominant constipation.

Q3.60
A. **False**
B. **True**
C. **False**
D. **True**
E. **False**
Neuroses are commonly found in irritable bowel syndrome and may respond to anxiolytics and antidepressants if symptoms are intractable.

Q3.61
A. **False**
B. **True**
C. **False**
D. **False**
E. **False**
This is not really a helpful diagnostic test as HLA B_8 is very common in the normal community.

Q3.62
A. **False**
B. **False**
C. **True**
D. **False**
E. **False**
The disease was paradoxically identified in Holland. There had been widespread starvation at the end of World War II, but children with coeliac disease appeared to do rather better. When wheat reappeared in the diet as a result of restored food supplies, coeliac children deteriorated sharply.

Q3.63
A. **False**
B. **False**
C. **True**
D. **False**
E. **False**
If IgA levels are raised lymphoma may have arisen.

Q3.64
A. True
B. False
C. True
D. True
E. True

Loss of gastric acid causes imbalance of the acid base system. Aspiration may cause pneumonitis. Mallory–Weiss tears may bleed, and actual rupture of the oesophagus can occur causing emphysema.

Q3.65
A. False
B. True
C. True
D. True
E. False

All of these have some role in protecting from coronary heart disease.

Q3.66
A. True
B. True
C. True
D. True
E. True

These general questions may well point to a diagnosis where more specific ones do not.

4. Large Bowel

Q4.1   Ischaemic colitis:

A. Is commoner in older patients
B. May present with painful bloody diarrhoea
C. Should be visible on flexible sigmoidoscopy
D. Has a specific histological appearance
E. Is usually associated with an abnormal ECG

Q4.2   If a patient with Crohn's disease presents with toxic dilatation of the colon:

A. Azathioprine and steroids will resolve the problem
B. The diagnosis may be really ulcerative colitis, and rectal biopsy may tell if so
C. Urgent colectomy may be required
D. Small bowel disease is always present
E. Bismuth chelate will destroy causative campylobacter

Q4.3   Active ulcerative colitis treated with the Truelove intensive intravenous regimen:

A. Usually eventually comes to surgery
B. May be managed with normal oral feeding
C. Requires steroid therapy
D. Should show some response within 5 days if the therapy is effective
E. May benefit from parenteral nutrition

Q4.4   The principle features which decide the prognosis in large bowel carcinoma are:

A. Age of patient
B. Site of tumour
C. Early diagnosis
D. Invasion through the serosa
E. Cigarette smoking

Q4.5   After total colectomy the following options are satisfactory in different patients:

A. Ileostomy
B. Ileorectal anastomosis
C. Re-epithelialisation of the rectum with small bowel mucosa
D. Ileal pouches
E. Ileal by-pass

Q4.6   What are the first-line treatments for ulcerative colitis:

A. Cyclophosphamide
B. Mesalazine
C. Topical steroids
D. Low roughage diet
E. Oral prednisolone

Q4.7   What is the active part of sulphasalazine:

A. Sulphapyramide
B. Sulphadimidine
C. Azathioprine
D. Aminosalicylate
E. Mesalazine

Q4.8   Sulphasalazine is definitely:

A. Useful in large bowel Crohn's disease
B. A cause of azoospermia
C. A cause of nausea and skin rashes
D. Cheaper than mesalazine
E. The cause of liver disease in ulcerative colitis

Q4.9   Treatment with mesalazine:

A. Should be lifelong in ulcerative colitis
B. Should be reserved for exacerbations
C. Is given in a standard maintenance dose of 6 g daily
D. May cause renal impairment
E. Can stain the fingers

Q4.10 Compared with steroid enemas in ulcerative colitis steroid foams are:

A. Much more effective
B. More effective
C. Equivalent
D. Less effective
E. Much less effective

Q4.11 In differentiating Crohn's disease from ulcerative colitis the following are useful pointers:

A. Severe abdominal pain unrelated to bowel action
B. Diarrhoea
C. Evidence of colonic involvement
D. Age at onset 20–40 years
E. Complications

Q4.12 Which of the following stimulate peristalsis:

A. Metoclopramide
B. Dicyclomine
C. Domperidone
D. Cisapride
E. Mebeverine

Q4.13 Which drugs inhibit peristalsis:

A. Atropine
B. Hyoscine butylbromide
C. Glucagon
D. Propantheline
E. Metoclopramide

Q4.14 Important peptide hormone synthesis and secretion occurs normally in:

A. The oesophagus
B. The stomach
C. The small bowel
D. The colon
E. The pancreas

Q4.15 The cells of the mucosa of the colon are:

A. Squamous
B. Keratinised
C. Transitional
D. Cuboidal
E. Columnar

Q4.16 *Entamoeba histolytica*:

A. Never occurs in Britain
B. Is still present in some former prisoners of World War II
C. Responds to metronidazole therapy
D. Causes liver abscesses
E. May be demonstrated in stool after provocative antibacterial therapy

Q4.17 A patient with a 30 mm polyp in the recto-sigmoid colon:

A. May be managed without open surgery
B. Always has positive stool occult blood tests
C. Requires full colonoscopy or barium enema
D. Probably has ulcerative colitis
E. Can be dealt with by biopsy and observation

Q4.18 Intestinal pseudo-obstruction:

A. Is usually spontaneous
B. Responds poorly to treatment
C. Can be managed by colonoscopy and flatus tubes
D. Is associated with hypokalaemia
E. May require caecostomy or ileo-rectal anastomosis

Q4.19 Flexible sigmoidoscopy:

A. Normally reaches the splenic flexure
B. Is more uncomfortable than rigid proctosigmoidoscopy
C. Often detects sigmoid abnormalities in diverticular disease
D. Replaces the need for barium enema
E. Requires in-patient preparation

Q4.20 The diarrhoea of ulcerative colitis may be effectively treated with:

A. Neomycin
B. Sulphadimidine
C. Codeine phosphate
D. Loperamide
E. Sulphasalazine

Q4.21 Normal stool frequency in Britain ranges between:

A. Once daily to once weekly
B. Twice daily to twice weekly
C. Thrice daily to thrice weekly
D. Four times daily to four times weekly
E. Five times daily to five times weekly

Q4.22 Histology of ulcerative colitis characteristically shows:

A. Goblet cell depletion
B. Transmural inflammation
C. Superficial ulceration
D. Crypt abscesses
E. String sign

Q4.23 At colonoscopy:

A. The distal rectum is not always seen well
B. The transverse colon has a triangular cross-section
C. The liver may be visible at the hepatic and splenic flexures
D. The caecum is wider than the rest of the bowel
E. Retrograde ileoscopy and ileography may be performed

Answers to Section 4

Q4.1
A. True
B. True
C. False
D. False
E. True
This condition predominantly affects the colon around the splenic flexure but is difficult to detect reliably on sigmoidoscopy. It is usually seen in elderly arteriopaths.

Q4.2
A. False
B. True
C. True
D. False
E. False
Toxic dilatation is an indication for early surgery if this can be safely performed. Diagnostic confusion is common in inflammatory bowel disease and evolving patterns may require changes in diagnosis between Crohn's disease and ulcerative colitis.

Q4.3
A. True
B. False
C. True
D. True
E. True
Vigorous intravenous treatment will improve most patients with active ulcerative colitis, but they frequently eventually do come to resection, even if this is an elective procedure in the future.

Q4.4
A. False
B. True
C. True
D. True
E. False
Early diagnosis will identify surgically curable tumours. Invasion through the serosa is Duke's C disease with a poor prognosis. Caecal carcinoma often presents late.

Q4.5
A. True
B. True
C. True
D. True
E. False

Modern restorative procedures have a place but patients must be prepared for conversion to ileostomy if they do not work well.

Q4.6
A. False
B. True
C. True
D. False
E. True

Azathioprine may have a reserve place in refractory disease.

Q4.7
A. False
B. False
C. False
D. True
E. False

It is local delivery of amino-salicylates which explains the activity of sulphasalazine.

Q4.8
A. True
B. True
C. True
D. True
E. False

10% of patients cannot take sulphasalazine and it is preferable to start new treatment courses with mesalazine.

Q4.9
A. True
B. False
C. False
D. True
E. False

Permanent treatment with mesalazine up to 2.5 g daily will reduce frequency and severity of exacerbations.

Q4.10
A. False
B. False
C. True
D. False
E. False

Patient preference determines whether foam or enemas are used.

Q4.11
A. True
B. False
C. False
D. False
E. True

Abdominal pain and perineal sepsis are typical of Crohn's disease.

Q4.12
A. True
B. False
C. True
D. True
E. False

These are the standard pro-kinetic agents. Mebeverine and dicyclomine are anti-spasmodics.

Q4.13
A. True
B. True
C. True
D. True
E. False

Parenteral treatment with atropinics or glucagon will promptly inhibit peristalsis.

Q4.14
A. False
B. True
C. True
D. False
E. True

Q4.15
A. False
B. False

C. **False**
D. **False**
E. **True**

The oesophagus and anus have squamous epithelium. The rest of the intestine is columnar.

Q4.16
A. **False**
B. **True**
C. **True**
D. **True**
E. **True**

Patients usually but not always give a history of travel abroad. Amoebas may be commensal in the homosexual bowel.

Q4.17
A. **True**
B. **False**
C. **True**
D. **False**
E. **False**

Sigmoidoscopic polypectomy may be all that is required, but the whole colon must be inspected to exclude other polyps or lesions.

Q4.18
A. **False**
B. **True**
C. **True**
D. **True**
E. **True**

Q4.19
A. **True**
B. **False**
C. **True**
D. **False**
E. **False**

Flexible sigmoidoscopy is much superior to rigid procto-sigmoidoscopy and should aim to reach the full length of the instrument, i.e. the splenic flexure and transverse colon. It is often required as a preliminary to barium enema to assess the proximal large bowel.

Q4.20
A. False
B. False
C. True
D. True
E. True

Anti-diarrhoeals and amino-salicylates are effective. Antibiotics may make the condition worse.

Q4.21
A. False
B. False
C. True
D. False
E. False

Change in bowel habit is often more important than absolute frequency.

Q4.22
A. True
B. False
C. True
D. True
E. False

These are the histological criteria of ulcerative colitis.

Q4.23
A. True
B. True
C. True
D. True
E. True

5. Liver and Spleen

Q5.1   Jaundice may be increased in Gilbert's syndrome by:

A. A glucose tolerance test
B. A high fat diet
C. Reduced energy intake
D. Intercurrent illness
E. Intravenous nicotinic acid

Q5.2   Jaundice in pregnancy is most likely to be caused by:

A. Bile duct stone
B. Benign intrahepatic cholestasis
C. Viral hepatitis
D. Pancreatitis
E. Carcinoma of the bile ducts

**Q5.3   A safe maximum limit for alcohol consumption in women below
          which physical harm does not occur is:**

A. 7 units/week
B. 14 units/week
C. 21 units/week
D. 28 units/week
E. 35 units/week

Q5.4   Since the 17th century alcohol consumption in Britain has:

A. Increased markedly
B. Increased a little
C. Stayed the same
D. Fallen a little
E. Fallen markedly

**Q5.5   A man who drinks 80 units of alcohol weekly for 10 years is at
          serious risk of:**

A. Chronic pancreatitis
B. Cerebral shrinkage
C. Impotence
D. Cirrhosis
E. Dyspepsia

Q5.6   The "CAGE" questionnaire enquires whether patients:

A. Have tried to *C*ut down alcohol intake
B. Have a good *A*ppetite
C. Feel *G*uilty about drinking
D. Have plenty of *E*nergy
E. Feel locked in

Q5.7   Alcoholism itself causes characteristic changes in:

A. Aspartate aminotransferase
B. Glutamyl transferase
C. Serum globulin
D. Red cell size
E. Erythrocyte sedimentation rate

Q5.8   Liver damage related to alcohol shows on biopsy as:

A. Steatosis
B. Hepatitis
C. Mallory's hyaline
D. Excess iron
E. Hepatoma

Q5.9   In alcoholic cirrhosis life may be prolonged by:

A. Stopping drinking alcohol
B. Colchicine
C. Prednisolone
D. Cyclosporin
E. Azathioprine

Q5.10 Primary biliary cirrhosis:

A. Is always cirrhotic on liver biopsy
B. Is always linked with mitochondrial antibody, titre 1/40+
C. Causes pruritus
D. Rarely causes symptoms
E. Rarely presents with jaundice

Q5.11 Infectious hepatitis:

A. Causes chronic liver disease
B. Causes gastroenteritis in children
C. Is followed by persistent IgG antibody and immunity
D. Is spread mainly by male homosexuals
E. Is often epidemic

Q5.12 Adult paracetamol overdose is managed by:

A. Oral activated charcoal
B. Ipecacuanha emesis
C. Liver transplantation
D. Routine acetylcysteine infusion
E. Measuring blood paracetamol, alanine aminotransferase and pro-
   thrombin ratio

Q5.13 Hepatitis B infection:

A. May be asymptomatic
B. Is only spread by blood transfusion
C. Causes liver cancer
D. Gives immunity to hepatitis A
E. Predisposes to delta hepatitis

Q5.14 Hepatitis B immunisation generally requires how many doses of
vaccine:

A. 1
B. 2
C. 3
D. 4
E. 5

Q5.15 Hepatitis non-A non-B infections:

A. Can be epidemic
B. Can be water-borne
C. Can follow blood transfusion
D. Can be detected by a specific serum antigen
E. Can be entirely excluded in a patient with a normal serum alanine
   aminotransferase and no hepatitis B surface antigen

Q5.16 Survival after liver transplant:

A. Levels off at about 70% after 1 year
B. Is better in black patients
C. Is better in children
D. Is better in primary biliary cirrhosis than in other diseases in adults
E. Is normal in hepatoma

Q5.17 A patient incidentally found to carry mitochondrial antibody:

A. Probably has primary biliary cirrhosis
B. May merely have thyrotoxicosis
C. Could have alcoholic liver disease
D. Must have a liver biopsy
E. Needs monthly clinic follow-up

Q5.18 In a patient with clotting disorder liver biopsy:

A. Is impossible
B. May be safe by the percutaneous routine with precautions
C. Can be performed with a trans-venous technique
D. Has frequently shown disease in haemophilia
E. Should be performed at laparotomy

Q5.19 Administration of nicotinic acid:

A. Induces haemolysis in G6PD deficiency
B. Causes flushing and diarrhoea
C. Induces jaundice in Gilbert's syndrome
D. Cures pellagra
E. Cures beri-beri

Q5.20 Early diagnosis of cholestatic jaundice is important because:

A. Bilirubin is toxic to adults
B. It clears hospital beds quickly
C. Incorrect management can be fatal
D. If surgery is needed it should be offered soon
E. Ultraviolet B therapy may be useful

Q5.21 A woman of 45 years with pruritus and no abnormality of serum biochemistry could have:

A. Polycythaemia rubra vera
B. Hodgkin's disease
C. Chronic active hepatitis
D. Primary biliary cirrhosis
E. Ankylosing spondylitis

Q5.22 Important histological findings in alcoholic liver disease include:

A. Councilman bodies
B. Excess iron deposition
C. Excess glycogen
D. Megamitchondria
E. Perivenular sclerosis

Q5.23 Which country has the highest individual alcohol intake:

A. Scotland
B. England
C. France
D. Italy
E. Iceland

Q5.24 What factors are important in governing national alcohol intake:

A. Religious beliefs
B. Cost
C. Wine-growing industry
D. Legislation
E. Political system of Government

Q5.25 Physical signs compatible with liver disease are:

A. Asterixis
B. Cyanosis
C. Clubbing
D. Testicular atrophy
E. Campbell de Morgan spots

Q5.26 Dupuytren's contracture:

A. Causes flexion deformity of the thumb
B. Can follow work with vibrating tools
C. Is seen in phenytoin therapy
D. May be familial
E. Suggests the cause of cirrhosis is alcohol

Q5.27 Hepatomegaly is defined as:

A. Enlargement of the liver above 1000 g
B. Displacement of the liver downwards
C. Presence of hepatic dullness at the costal margin
D. Palpability of the liver edge several centimetres below the rib margin, where the upper border can be percussed above the level of the nipple
E. Presence of abnormal deposits of fat, glycogen or iron

Q5.28 The spleen enlarges:

A. Towards the left iliac fossa
B. Towards the right iliac fossa
C. Towards the right upper quadrant
D. Posteriorly
E. Anteriorly

Q5.29 The notch of the spleen lies:

A. Superiorly
B. Inferiorly
C. Anterior and medially
D. Posteriorly
E. Laterally

Q5.30 In Africa the commonest form of hepatitis is:

A. Bush tea drinking
B. Delta virus
C. Alcoholism
D. Hepatitis B
E. AIDS

Q5.31 The pyrrolizidine in certain herbs is dangerous because it causes hepatic:

A. Steatosis
B. Granulomas
C. Bile duct destruction
D. Veno-occlusive disease
E. Pigmentation

Q5.32 Bleeding disorders in liver disease are caused by deficiency in:

A. Factor II
B. Factor VII
C. Factor X
D. Vitamin K
E. Platelets

Q5.33 Hepatic encephalopathy causes:

A. Flapping tremor
B. Pill-rolling tremor
C. Intention tremor
D. EEG delta waves
E. Proptosis

Q5.34 Important mechanisms in ascites include:

A. Renal water retention
B. Low body sodium
C. Portal hypertension
D. Hypoalbuminaemia
E. Oestrogen excess

Q5.35 Alcoholic cirrhosis may be associated with:

A. Obesity
B. Cachexia
C. Prolonged life expectancy because of raised HDL-2 cholesterol levels
D. Improved prognosis if nourishing stout is drunk instead of spirits
E. Scurvy

Q5.36 In chronic auto-immune hepatitis the following are characteristically present:

A. Mitochondrial antibody
B. Gliadin antibody
C. Nuclear antibody
D. α-1-antitrypsin deficiency
E. Smooth muscle antibody

Q5.37 Wilson's disease is:

A. Hepatolenticular degeneration
B. Familial
C. Associated with corneal arcus
D. The only cause of excess hepatic copper
E. Common

Q5.38 The most useful tests in haemochromatosis include:

A. Haemoglobin level
B. Serum iron
C. Serum ferritin
D. Liver biopsy
E. Urine iron excretion after desferrioxamine

Q5.39 Venesection is useful in:

A. Polycythaemia
B. Porphyria
C. Thrombocytopenia
D. Leukaemia
E. Haemochromatosis

Q5.40 Which organisms are specially prone to cause liver damage:

A. *Diphyllobothrium latum*
B. *Entamoeba histolytica*
C. *Plasmodium vivax*
D. *Schistosoma mansonii*
E. *Clonorchis sinesis*

Q5.41 Herald symptoms in primary biliary cirrhosis are:

A. Jaundice
B. Pruritus
C. Lethargy
D. Caput medusae
E. Ascites

Q5.42 The following improve survival in cirrhosis:

A. Frusemide
B. Lactulose
C. Multi-vitamins
D. Chlormethiazole
E. Paracentesis

Q5.43 The spleen is:

A. Particularly vulnerable to trauma
B. Sometimes ruptured in infectious mononucleosis
C. Sometimes accompanied by accessory spleens
D. Always removed at gastroscopy
E. Protective against pneumococcal infections

Q5.44 The following viruses cause hepatitis:

A. Ebola fever
B. Marburg disease
C. Bornholm disease
D. Epstein–Barr virus
E. Cytomegalovirus

Q5.45 Non-infective causes of fatty liver include:

A. Diabetes mellitus
B. High cholesterol diet
C. Malnutrition
D. Morbid obesity
E. Drinking carbon tetrachloride

Q5.46 The normal liver in life is most nearly described as coloured:

A. Green
B. Yellow
C. Crimson
D. Brown
E. Black

Q5.47 For bleeding oesophageal varices what options are useful:

A. Vagotomy and pyloroplasty
B. Total gastrectomy
C. Highly selective vagotomy
D. Spleno-renal venous anastomosis
E. Oesophageal transection

Q5.48 Adverse reactions affecting the liver are characteristically seen with:

A. Cephalosporins
B. Fusidic acid
C. Erythromycin
D. Pencillins
E. Aminoglycosides

Q5.49 Methyldopa has been implicated in:

A. Haemolytic anaemia
B. Sclerosing cholangitis
C. Chronic active hepatitis
D. Lupoid syndrome
E. Polyarteritis nodosa

Q5.50 The following tests are characteristically abnormal in cholestatic liver disease:

A. IgA
B. IgD
C. IgE
D. IgG
E. IgM

Q5.51 Raised blood cholesterol in cholestatic liver disease is linked to elevation of:

A. Apolipoprotein AI
B. Apolipoprotein AII
C. Apolipoprotein B
D. Apolipoprotein C
E. Apolipoprotein X

Q5.52 What metals are causes of cirrhosis:

A. Lead
B. Manganese
C. Copper
D. Gold
E. Iron

Q5.53 Ascites in cirrhosis may be managed by:

A. Paracentesis
B. Frusemide
C. Ethacrynic acid
D. Low protein diet
E. Amiloride

Q5.54 Hyponatraemia in liver disease:

A. Is frequently refractory
B. Responds to water deprivation
C. Is treated by oral sodium chloride
D. Only improves with intravenous saline
E. Indicates that diuretic therapy is useless

Q5.55 α-1-antitrypsin deficiency causes:

A. Emphysema
B. Asthma
C. Pulmonary oedema
D. Hepatitis in adults
E. Cirrhosis

Q5.56 In schistosomiasis the following are seen:

A. Obstructive jaundice
B. Portal hypertension
C. Hyposplenism
D. Pancreatitis
E. Ulcerative jejunoileitis

Q5.57 The presence of liver metastases:

A. Is sometimes shown by raised carcinoembryonic antigen
B. Will show on ultrasonography when deposits are greater than 10 mm
C. Shows as "hot" areas on isotope scanning
D. Causes raised alkaline phosphatase
E. Causes hypoalbuminaemia

Q5.58 Liver abscess occur in:

A. Inflammatory bowel disease
B. Amoebiasis
C. Congestive cardiac failure
D. Coeliac disease
E. Zollinger–Ellison syndrome

Q5.59 In congestive cardiac failure with cirrhosis:

A. The cause is digoxin therapy
B. Diuretic therapy is less effective in controlling ascites
C. The cause is auto-immune
D. Cyclophosphamide may be useful
E. The "nutmeg" liver is seen

Q5.60 Hepatosplenomegaly is a sign in:

A. β-Thalassaemia
B. Hodgkin's disease
C. Amyloidosis
D. Portal hypertension
E. Acute myeloid leukaemia

Q5.61 Chronic liver disease is accompanied by:

A. Anaemia
B. Polycythaemia
C. Uraemia
D. Low serum urea
E. Hyperkalaemia

Q5.62 Diseases of the liver and pancreas are sometimes associated because:

A. They have the same blood supply
B. Diabetes can damage the liver
C. Cirrhosis damages the pancreas
D. Alcohol damages both organs
E. They are close together

Q5.63 In normal liver sinusoids the following are present:

A. Kupffer cells
B. Parenchymal cells
C. Fibrocytes
D. Ito cells
E. Endothelial cells

Q5.64 Cirrhosis is defined as:

A. Hepatic steatosis
B. Hepatic inflammation
C. Hepatic necrosis and regeneration
D. Hepatic hypertrophy
E. Kupffer cell dysfunction

Q5.65 Special histological stains for iron in haemochromatosis include:

A. Perl's reagent
B. Mallory's hyaline
C. Masson's trichrome
D. Haemotoxylin and eosin
E. Reticulin stain

Q5.66 Thrombus in the venules on liver histology is seen in:

A. Portal hypertension
B. Obstructive jaundice
C. Bush tea drinkers
D. Fatty liver
E. Banti's syndrome

Q5.67 In cholestatic jaundice if the ultrasonogram shows dilated ducts:

A. Gallstones may be the cause
B. PTC invariably succeeds
C. ERCP may fail because of ampullary tumours
D. Observation is useful
E. Liver failure may be expected

Q5.68 The damage caused by paracetamol overdose to the liver can be prevented by:

A. Monosodium glutamate
B. Methionine
C. Alcohol
D. Cysteamine
E. Acetylcysteine

Q5.69 Liver failure results in bleeding:

A. From erosions
B. Because of thrombocytopenia
C. Because of vitamin E deficiency
D. Because of complex clotting abnormality
E. Which can be prevented by ranitidine IV

Q5.70 In hepatic encephalopathy the following are useful:

A. High protein diet
B. Neomycin intravenously
C. Lactose
D. Twice normal saline infusion with added potassium
E. Chlorpromazine

Q5.71 The normal time taken to complete a trail test with 25 points is:

A. 10 seconds
B. 20 seconds
C. 30 seconds
D. 60 seconds
E. 90 seconds

Q5.72 The following drugs are known to cause liver damage on occasions:

A. Chlorpromazine
B. Cimetidine
C. Clofibrate
D. Colestipol
E. Cholecystokinin

Q5.73 Modern effective treatments for liver failure include:

A. Transplantation
B. Exchange transfusion
C. Charcoal haemoperfusion
D. Electroconvulsive therapy
E. Oral diazepam

Q5.74 The complication rate in percutaneous liver biopsy relates to:

A. Biliary obstruction
B. Ascites
C. Prothrombin ratio
D. Number of punctures
E. Fatty liver

Q5.75 Hepatoma is treated by:

A. Portal vein litigation
B. Bleomycin
C. Daunorubicin
D. Liver transplantation
E. α-Fetoprotein

Q5.76 Enlargement of the spleen is detected in:

A. Coeliac disease
B. Diverticular disease
C. Haemolysis
D. Portal hypertension
E. Acute pancreatitis

Q5.77 In viral hepatitis:

A. There are good serum markers for all types
B. α-Interferon may be useful in chronic hepatitis B
C. Steroids only benefit cholestasis
D. Active immunisation is useful for hepatitis B prevention
E. Presence of HB_eAg is an important indicator of infectivity

Q5.78 Jaundice may be seen in:

A. Haemolytic anaemia
B. Crigler–Najjar syndrome
C. Mepacrine therapy
D. Dietary carrot excess
E. Cholecystolithiasis

Q5.79 Isotope scanning with hepatic iminodiacetic acid (HIDA) derivatives:

A. Shows liver metastases
B. Outlines gallstones
C. Shows a non-functioning gallbladder in acute cholecystitis
D. Will show delayed or absent excretion into the small intestine in extra-hepatic obstruction
E. Depends on liver blood flow

Q5.80 Elevation of alkaline phosphatase and glutamyl transferase without jaundice is seen in:

A. Hepatitis C
B. Gallstones
C. Primary biliary cirrhosis
D. Liver metastases
E. Paget's disease

Answers to Section 5

Q5.1
A. False
B. False
C. True
D. True
E. True
Increase of serum bilirubin by at least 50% on a reduced energy diet for 48 hours is a useful diagnostic test.

Q5.2
A. False
B. True
C. True
D. False
E. False
These are the 2 commonest causes of jaundice in pregnancy, though all the options are possible.

Q5.3
A. False
B. False
C. True
D. False
E. False
This was the official Government recommendation in 1995.

Q5.4
A. False
B. False
C. False
D. False
E. True
The moderate increase since 1950 is much less impressive than the continuous decline in the previous 2½ centuries.

Q5.5
A. True
B. True
C. True
D. True
E. True
This is alcoholism.

Q5.6
A. True
B. False
C. True
D. False
E. False
(A) is asking about Annoyance of criticism of drinking
(E) is taking an Eye-opener drink to start the day

Q5.7
A. True
B. True
C. False
D. True
E. False
These are useful but not invariable clues.

Q5.8
A. True
B. True
C. True
D. True
E. True
The presence of hepatitis is even more important than of cirrhosis in predicting outcome. Hepatoma will be a terminal event.

Q5.9
A. True
B. True
C. False
D. False
E. False
Prednisolone treatment in alcoholic hepatitis remains contentious.

Q5.10
A. **False**
B. **False**
C. **True**
D. **False**
E. **True**

Though primary biliary cirrhosis may be symptomatic, it commonly presents with pruritus and lethargy. Jaundice is a late feature.

Q5.11
A. **False**
B. **True**
C. **True**
D. **False**
E. **True**

Hepatitis A never causes chronic liver disease and is transmitted by the faecal-oral route.

Q5.12
A. **True**
B. **False**
C. **True**
D. **False**
E. **True**

Activated charcoal will reduce absorption and liver transplantation may be required in the minority where intractable liver failure develops. Acetyl-cysteine should be reserved for patients who have definitely taken more than 15 g of paracetamol (7.5 g in alcoholics), or where plasma paracetamol levels after 4 hours indicate the necessity.

Q5.13
A. **True**
B. **False**
C. **True**
D. **False**
E. **True**

Asymptomatic carriers may be the cause of infection. Screening of blood for transfusion means this is not an important route of transmission now. Hepatitis B may eventually lead to hepatoma. The hepatitis D virus can only afflict people already infected with hepatitis B.

Q5.14
A. **False**
B. **False**

C. True
D. False
E. False
Two initial immunisations a month apart and a booster are probably sufficient.

Q5.15
A. True
B. True
C. True
D. False
E. False
Mostly these are hepatitis C and E but there are also other viruses, e.g. HGV.

Q5.16
A. True
B. False
C. True
D. True
E. False

Q5.17
A. True
B. False
C. True
D. False
E. False
Mitochondrial antibody to a titre of greater than 40, and especially the presence of the M2 sub-fraction, are very strongly linked with primary biliary cirrhosis; but these patients are not protected from alcoholic liver disease if they drink.

Q5.18
A. False
B. True
C. True
D. True
E. False
Many patients with haemophilia are affected by hepatitis C. Transvenous biopsy is safe but often yields disappointingly small samples. Percutaneous or laparoscopic biopsies taken after appropriate transfusions of fresh frozen plasma and platelets make most patients biopsiable.

Q5.19
A. **False**
B. **True**
C. **True**
D. **True**
E. **False**

The best use of nicotinic acid is in curing pellagra. Unacceptably toxic doses are required in hypercholesterolaemia and there are usually better alternatives.

Q5.20
A. **False**
B. **False**
C. **True**
D. **True**
E. **False**

The major differential is between extrahepatic obstruction which will require surgical or endoscopic management, and intrahepatic cholestasis where surgery is hazardous.

Q5.21
A. **True**
B. **True**
C. **False**
D. **True**
E. **False**

Many cases of skin itching have no definite cause, or a dermatological explanation.

Q5.22
A. **False**
B. **True**
C. **False**
D. **True**
E. **True**

The presence of peri-venular sclerosis has adverse prognostic significance.

Q5.23
A. **False**
B. **False**
C. **False**
D. **False**

E. True
It is worth noting that Scotland, France and Italy are all well ahead of
England too.

Q5.24
A. True
B. True
C. True
D. True
E. False

Q5.25
A. True
B. False
C. True
D. True
E. False
Campbell de Morgan spots have no diagnostic significance and cyanosis is
not a feature of liver disease. Asterixis is a flapping tremor. Testicular
atrophy occurs because of altered steroid hormone metabolism.

Q5.26
A. False
B. True
C. True
D. True
E. True
This condition is often idiopathic and causes flexion deformity of the ring
and little fingers.

Q5.27
A. False
B. False
C. False
D. True
E. False

Q5.28
A. False
B. True
C. False
D. False

E.   False
Gross enlargement of the spleen may be missed unless the examination is commenced in the right lower quadrant.

Q5.29
A. False
B. False
C. True
D. False
E. False

Q5.30
A. False
B. False
C. False
D. True
E. False
B virus infection is very common in developing countries.

Q5.31
A. False
B. False
C. False
D. True
E. False
This may be important because leaves used in herb tea may contain these toxins.

Q5.32
A. True
B. True
C. True
D. True
E. True
Haemorrhage is usually multifactorial.

Q5.33
A. True
B. False
C. False
D. True

E. False

Pill-rolling tremor is seen in Parkinsonism, intention tremor in cerebellar disease, and proptosis is a hallmark of thyrotoxicosis.

Q5.34

A. True
B. False
C. True
D. True
E. False

Body sodium is usually raised in liver disease causing ascites though serum levels may be low.

Q5.35

A. True
B. True
C. False
D. False
E. True

Alcoholics are usually malnourished in some way though the patterns are variable.

Q5.36

A. False
B. False
C. True
D. False
E. True

This is the classic pattern of chronic auto-immune hepatitis. Variants may carry different antibodies, such as LKM microsomal antibody.

Q5.37

A. True
B. True
C. False
D. False
E. False

Wilson's disease is uncommon and strongly familial. Copper deposition may be associated with other illnesses such as primary biliary cirrhosis where its significance is uncertain.

Q5.38
A. False
B. True
C. True
D. True
E. True
Hb. level is often quite normal.

Q5.39
A. True
B. True
C. False
D. False
E. True

Q5.40
A. False
B. True
C. True
D. True
E. True
The fish tape worm does not affect the liver.

Q5.41
A. False
B. True
C. True
D. False
E. False
The development of liver failure is a late feature in the disease.

Q5.42
A. False
B. False
C. False
D. False
E. False
Though all of these treatments may be appropriate none is shown to improve longevity.

Q5.43
A. True
B. True
C. True
D. False
E. True
Preservation of the spleen at abdominal surgery is worthwhile if possible.

Q5.44
A. True
B. True
C. False
D. True
E. True
Bornholm disease is intercostal myalgia.

Q5.45
A. True
B. False
C. True
D. True
E. False

Q5.46
A. False
B. False
C. True
D. False
E. False

Q5.47
A. False
B. False
C. False
D. True
E. True
Injection sclerotherapy, banding, and treatment with propranolol, somato-statin and nitrates have also been used.

Q5.48
A. False
B. True

C. **True**
D. **False**
E. **False**

Q5.49
A. **True**
B. **False**
C. **True**
D. **True**
E. **False**
Adverse reactions have been largely responsible for the diminished usage of this antihypertensive drug.

Q5.50
A. **False**
B. **False**
C. **False**
D. **True**
E. **True**
These are characteristically raised in auto-immune liver disease.

Q5.51
A. **False**
B. **False**
C. **False**
D. **False**
E. **True**
High cholesterol levels in cholestatic liver disease do not appear to be linked with increased risk of heart disease.

Q5.52
A. **False**
B. **False**
C. **True**
D. **False**
E. **True**
These are Wilson's disease and haemochromatosis.

Q5.53
A. **True**
B. **True**
C. **True**

D. **False**
E. **True**

Low protein diet may benefit encephalopathy but will not improve ascites.

Q5.54

A. **True**
B. **False**
C. **False**
D. **False**
E. **False**

Hyponatraemia does not necessarily have adverse effects and is not usually an indication for treatment.

Q5.55

A. **True**
B. **False**
C. **False**
D. **False**
E. **True**

It is often different patients who develop the lung or liver disease.

Q5.56

A. **False**
B. **True**
C. **False**
D. **False**
E. **False**

Q5.57

A. **True**
B. **True**
C. **False**
D. **True**
E. **False**

No test is completely reliable in excluding small liver metastases. MRI scanning has been suggested as the best anatomical test.

Q5.58

A. **True**
B. **True**
C. **False**
D. **False**
E. **False**

Portal sepsis explains liver abscesses in inflammatory bowel disease, whereas direct amoebic infection occurs in amoebiasis.

Q5.59
A. **False**
B. **True**
C. **False**
D. **False**
E. **True**

When heart failure has caused liver disease fluid retention becomes multi-factorial.

Q5.60
A. **True**
B. **True**
C. **True**
D. **True**
E. **False**

Acute myeloid leukaemia would not affect the liver.

Q5.61
A. **True**
B. **True**
C. **True**
D. **True**
E. **False**

Hypokalaemia is more characteristic of chronic liver disease because of aldosteronism.

Q5.62
A. **False**
B. **True**
C. **False**
D. **True**
E. **False**

Q5.63
A. **True**
B. **False**
C. **False**
D. **True**
E. **True**

Parenchymal cells are not found in the sinusoids. If fibrocytes occur this would be pathological and suggestive of developing cirrhosis.

Q5.64
A. False
B. False
C. True
D. False
E. False

Q5.65
A. True
B. False
C. False
D. False
E. False

This gives a vivid blue colour when iron is present and the pattern of deposition will indicate whether haemochromatosis is present.

Q5.66
A. False
B. False
C. True
D. False
E. True

Q5.67
A. True
B. True
C. True
D. False
E. True

Extra-hepatic obstruction requires early accurate diagnosis and treatment to avoid morbidity and mortality.

Q5.68
A. False
B. True
C. False
D. True
E. True

Only intravenous acetylcysteine and oral methionine are used in standard therapy now.

Q5.69
A. True
B. True
C. False
D. True
E. True
Vitamin K deficiency may contribute to bleeding liver failure.

Q5.70
A. False
B. False
C. False
D. False
E. False
None of these will work, and chlorpromazine will make the patient worse.

Q5.71
A. False
B. False
C. True
D. False
E. False
This is a useful quantitative test of development and regression of hepatic encephalopathy.

Q5.72
A. True
B. True
C. False
D. False
E. False

Q5.73
A. True
B. False
C. True
D. False
E. False

Q5.74
A. True
B. True
C. True

D. True
E. False

Q5.75
A. False
B. False
C. True
D. True
E. False

Regrettably neither chemotherapy nor liver transplantation for tumours over 3 cm diameter are very effective.

Q5.76
A. False
B. False
C. True
D. True
E. False

Coeliac disease causes hyposplenism.

Q5.77
A. False
B. True
C. True
D. True
E. True

Most common viral hepatitis can be diagnosed by serum markers, but some varieties cannot.

Q5.78
A. True
B. True
C. True
D. True
E. True

Q5.79
A. False
B. False
C. True
D. True
E. False

This is a useful technique for diagnosing acute cholecystitis if it can be performed early in the illness.

Q5.80
A. **False**
B. **True**
C. **True**
D. **True**
E. **False**

In Paget's disease alkaline phosphatase is elevated but not glutamyl transferase, and in hepatitis C serum bilirubin and transaminase are characteristically elevated.

6. Pancreas and Gallbladder

Q6.1 Pancreatic carcinoma is:

A. Becoming commoner
B. Related to alcohol abuse
C. Related to cigarette smoking
D. 98% fatal in 5 years
E. Excluded by normal endoscopic pancreatography

Q6.2 Causes of acute pancreatitis are:

A. Duodenal ulcers
B. Gallstone disease
C. Alcoholism
D. Progesterone therapy
E. Laparotomy

Q6.3 Chronic pancreatitis is diagnosed by:

A. Pentagastrin test
B. Lundh test
C. Secretin test
D. Bentiromide test
E. Fluorescein dilaurate test

Q6.4 Cancer of the pancreas presents as:

A. Jaundice
B. Pain
C. Diabetes mellitus
D. Fluctuating bluish skin rash
E. Diarrhoea

Q6.5 The secretions of the pancreas are:

A. Acidic to help protein digestion
B. Alkaline to neutralise gastric acid
C. Mainly zymogens
D. Increased by cholecystokinin
E. Increased by secretin

Q6.6 Chronic pancreatitis is frequently:

A. A cause of severe steatorrhoea
B. Idiopathic
C. Related to gallstone disease
D. Alcoholic
E. Painless

Q6.7 Pancreatic enzymes which can usefully be demonstrated in the serum are:

A. Trypsin
B. Chymotrypsin
C. Amylase
D. Enterokinase
E. Lipase

Q6.8 Screening for cystic fibrosis depends on:

A. Nappy trypsin levels
B. Sputum microbiology
C. Low sweat chloride
D. High sweat sodium
E. Dried blood spot trypsin levels

Q6.9 Treatments which may be helpful in pancreatic insufficiency are:

A. Pancreatin
B. Low fat diet
C. Steroids
D. Cholecystectomy
E. Exchange transfusion

Q6.10 Tests which are very useful in pancreatic disease include:

A. Barium meal
B. Small bowel enema
C. Retrograde pancreatography
D. Retrograde cholangiography
E. Computed tomography

Q6.11 Drugs plausibly linked to acute pancreatitis are:

A. Prednisolone
B. Oral contraceptives
C. Chlorpromazine
D. Clofibrate
E. Cholestyramine

Q6.12 A patient with severe abdominal pain and jaundice may have:

A. Uncomplicated acute pancreatitis
B. Uncomplicated acute cholecystitis
C. Common bile duct stones
D. Gallstones and acute pancreatitis
E. Chronic pancreatitis and carcinoma of the pancreas

Q6.13 Gallbladder cancer is:

A. A disease of advancing age
B. Generally seen in non-functioning gallbladders
C. Incurable if more than very early
D. Associated with gallstones
E. Diagnosed by histology after elective cholecystectomy on occasions

Q6.14 Mortality after planned cholecystectomy in a 40-year-old should be:

A. Less than 1%
B. 1%
C. 1.5%
D. 2%
E. 2.5%

Q6.15 Factors which lead to worsening results after gallbladder surgery are:

A. Female sex
B. Oral contraceptive use
C. Age 60+ years
D. Presence of bile duct stones
E. Numerous gallbladder stones

Q6.16 Gallstones can be dissolved by:

A. Lithocholic acid
B. Cholic acid
C. Deoxycholic acid
D. Chenodeoxycholic acid
E. Ursodeoxycholic acid

Q6.17 Complications of dissolution treatment are:

A. Induced calcification of stones
B. Low overall efficacy
C. Need to select cases
D. Substantial recurrence risk
E. Prolonged therapy

Q6.18 Bile acids are also useful in:

A. Dyspepsia
B. Primary biliary cirrhosis
C. Cerebrotendinous xanthomatosis
D. Chronic active hepatitis
E. *Clonorchis sinesis* infection

Q6.19 Options available for radiopaque gallstones are:

A. Oral dissolution
B. Surgical removal
C. Methyltertiary butyl ether
D. Lithotripsy
E. Percutaneous cholecystectomy

Q6.20 Gallstones show on plain radiography if there is:

A. High cholesterol content
B. Mercedes-Benz sign
C. Ring clarification
D. Phrygian cap
E. Functioning gallbladder

Q6.21 Common bile duct stones:

A. Are often associated with cholecystolithiasis
B. Are well demonstrated in cholecystography
C. Can be a cause of acute pancreatitis
D. Can be removed at ERCP
E. Cause Mirizzi syndrome

Q6.22 Analysis of duodenal bile:

A. Shows microspheroliths with pigment stones
B. Is routine in diagnosis
C. Shows crystals with cholesterol stones
D. Does not always produce accurate results because of dilution
E. Predicts stone disease from cholesterol saturation in individuals

Q6.23 Pancreozymin is also known as:

A. Ceruletide
B. Caeruloplasmin
C. Octapeptide
D. Cholecystokinin
E. Prostacyclin

Q6.24 Acute acalculous cholecystitis:

A. Is seen after abdominal surgery
B. Is harmless
C. Can be associated with gallbladder gas
D. Means biliary dyskinesia
E. Requires surgical treatment usually

Q6.25 The highest frequency of gallstones is seen in:

A. Bangladesh
B. India
C. Pakistan
D. Red Indians
E. Afghanistan

Q6.26 The lowest prevalence of gallstones occurs in:

A. South Africa
B. Japan
C. Zambia
D. Australia
E. Florida

Q6.27 Gallstones are rich in:

A. Bile acids
B. Lecithin
C. Cholesterol
D. Bilirubin
E. Calcium salts

Q6.28 Major risk for gallstones include:

A. Female sex
B. Advancing age
C. Fibric acid drugs
D. Haemolysis
E. Race

Q6.29 Gallstones cause symptoms:

A. Always
B. Usually
C. Sometimes
D. Rarely
E. Never

Q6.30 Gallstones are associated with:

A. Gallbladder carcinoma
B. Hypercholesterolaemia
C. Cholesterolosis
D. Aschoff–Rokitansky sinuses
E. Biliary dyskinesia

Q6.31 The best test for gallstone disease is:

A. Symptomatology
B. Physical examination
C. Abdominal X-Ray
D. Cholecystography
E. Ultrasonography

Q6.32 In children pancreatic insufficiency is caused by:

A. Schwachman–Diamond syndrome
B. Familial calcific pancreatitis
C. Glucagonoma
D. Cystic fibrosis
E. Haemolytic anaemia

Q6.33 Survival in cystic fibrosis:

A. Has a median in the late teens
B. Depends on pancreatic disease
C. Is longer in males
D. Depends on parental social class
E. Is much longer than 30 years ago

Q6.34 Autosomal recessive disorders amenable to control by carrier detection include:

A. Crohn's disease
B. Coeliac disease
C. α_1-Antitrypsin deficiency
D. Cystic fibrosis
E. Sickle cell disease

Q6.35 Chronic pancreatitis can be detected by:

A. Calcification on radiology
B. Low duodenal bicarbonate after secretin stimulation
C. Impaired fluorescein excretion after oral fluorescein dilaurate
D. Low serum and urine PABA after oral betiromide
E. Retrograde pancreatography

Q6.36 Pseudocyst formation:

A. Means retrograde pancreatography is best deferred
B. Occurs in cystic fibrosis
C. Is frequent in haemochromatosis
D. Is treated by cyanoacrylate injection
E. Is detected by ultrasonography

Answers to Section 6

Q6.1
A. True
B. True
C. True
D. True
E. False
This condition may be very difficult to diagnose whatever tests are used. The serum marker CA 19-9 may be raised and is a fairly specific marker.

Q6.2
A. True
B. True
C. True
D. False
E. True
Acute pancreatitis is commonly related to gallstones in women and alcoholism in men, but the next major group is idiopathic.

Q6.3
A. False
B. True
C. True
D. True
E. True
All these tests detect pancreatic enzymes whereas the pentagastrin test measures gastric acid after stimulation.

Q6.4
A. True
B. True
C. True
D. False
E. True
The fluctuating bluish skin rash is a feature of glucagonoma.

Q6.5
A. False
B. True
C. True
D. True
E. True

Q6.6
A. True
B. True
C. False
D. True
E. False
Though gallstone disease may be seen in chronic pancreatitis it is probably an incidental. The condition is usually painful.

Q6.7
A. True
B. False
C. True
D. False
E. True
In practice amylase is the only freely available enzyme test.

Q6.8
A. False
B. False
C. False
D. True
E. True
Genetic screening may also be useful.

Q6.9
A. True
B. True
C. False
D. False
E. False
It is better to use pancreatic extracts to preserve nutrition, though a low fat diet may be required if steatorrhoea is intractable otherwise.

Q6.10
A. **False**
B. **False**
C. **True**
D. **True**
E. **True**
Acute pancreatitis may be associated with bile duct stones.

Q6.11
A. **True**
B. **True**
C. **False**
D. **True**
E. **False**
Many other associations have been postulated.

Q6.12
A. **True**
B. **True**
C. **True**
D. **True**
E. **True**
Diagnosis is not always easy!

Q6.13
A. **True**
B. **True**
C. **True**
D. **True**
E. **True**
Fortunately this condition is not common as it is very difficult to diagnose
and treat.

Q6.14
A. **True**
B. **False**
C. **False**
D. **False**
E. **False**
Mortality is lower after laparoscopic cholecystectomy than open cholecys-
tectomy.

Q6.15
A. False
B. False
C. True
D. True
E. False

Q6.16
A. False
B. False
C. False
D. True
E. True

The place of dissolution therapy is small but it has a role in patients who refuse or are unsuitable for surgery.

Q6.17
A. True
B. True
C. True
D. True
E. True

These drawbacks limit the usefulness of therapy.

Q6.18
A. True
B. True
C. True
D. True
E. False

It is only in primary biliary cirrhosis and primary sclerosing cholangitis that ursodeoxycholic acid therapy has established a routine therapeutic place.

Q6.19
A. False
B. True
C. False
D. True
E. True

Cholecystectomy and endoscopic removal are the best options where feasible.

Q6.20
A. False
B. True
C. True
D. False
E. False

The Mercedes-Benz sign is caused by gas filled fractures in stones. Ring calcification occurs because of deposition of calcium in layers on the periphery of the growing stone.

Q6.21
A. True
B. False
C. True
D. True
E. False

Mirizzi syndrome is caused by gallbladder stones and cholangiography is usually necessary to show bile duct stones.

Q6.22
A. True
B. False
C. True
D. True
E. False

This is not a standard diagnostic technique but can sometimes be useful.

Q6.23
A. False
B. False
C. False
D. True
E. False

Q6.24
A. True
B. False
C. True
D. False
E. True

Patients are often very severely unwell with this condition.

Q6.25

A. **False**
B. **False**
C. **False**
D. **True**
E. **False**

Various tribes have been studied and they all seem to hold the world record.

Q6.26

A. **False**
B. **False**
C. **True**
D. **False**
E. **False**

Cholesterol gallstones seem to be a problem of developed countries and modern diet trends.

Q6.27

A. **False**
B. **False**
C. **True**
D. **True**
E. **True**

These are the principal components of most gallstones. Bile acids and lecithin are usually confined to the bile.

Q6.28

A. **True**
B. **True**
C. **True**
D. **True**
E. **True**

Q6.29

A. **False**
B. **False**
C. **True**
D. **False**
E. **False**

Most gallstones are asymptomatic.

Q6.30
A. True
B. False
C. False
D. False
E. False

This association is mostly of significance in Red Indians where prophylactic cholecystectomy may be useful. It is not considered important for other groups.

Q6.31
A. False
B. False
C. False
D. False
E. True

Most gallstones are found in the gallbladder and ultrasonography is the best way of detecting them.

Q6.32
A. True
B. True
C. False
D. True
E. False

Schwachman–Diamond syndrome is notable for fluctuating neutropenia. Calcific pancreatitis can be diagnosed by family history and X-Ray. Cystic fibrosis can be shown by sweat testing and genetic screening.

Q6.33
A. True
B. False
C. True
D. True
E. True

Lung disease is the main predictor of longevity.

Q6.34
A. False
B. False
C. True
D. True
E. True

Q6.35
A. **True**
B. **True**
C. **True**
D. **True**
E. **True**

Q6.36
A. **False**
B. **False**
C. **False**
D. **False**
E. **True**
Though best detected by ultrasound examination, pseudocysts may require retrograde pancreatography for full definition, and this appears to be safe.